# Questions and Answers in MEDICINE FOR STUDENTS

## B. T. COOPER MD MRCP
*Lecturer in Medicine*

and

## M. J. HALL MB MRCP
*Lecturer in Medicine*
*University Department of Medicine,*
*Bristol Royal Infirmary,*
*Bristol*

## WRIGHT

Bristol
1984

*Published by:*
John Wright & Sons Ltd, Techno House, Redcliffe Way, Bristol BS1 6NX, England


*First Published,* 1984
*Reprinted,* 1985

*British Library Cataloguing in Publication Data*

Cooper, B. T.
  Questions and answers in medicine for students.
  1. Medicine—Problems, exercises, etc.
  I. Title    II. Hall, M. J.
  610'.76    R834.5


ISBN 0 7236 0686 2


Library of Congress Catalog Card Number: 83–57405


Typeset by Severntype Repro Services Ltd and printed and bound
in Great Britain by John Wright & Sons (Printing) Ltd. at The Stonebridge Press,
Bristol BS4 5NU

# *Preface*

This book is aimed primarily at undergraduates about to sit their final examinations in medicine although candidates for higher examinations in medicine may find it useful. The book is a companion volume to *Questions and Answers in Surgery for Students* by Kelly, Kelly and Henderson and its format and its aims are the same. Not only does this book seek to provide a relatively simple and straightforward method of revision and self-assessment for those sitting final examinations, but it also aims to provide some of the knowledge which the newly-qualified doctor needs on the wards and in the casualty department. Hence many of the questions are about the practicalities of management of emergencies or of acute and difficult situations which the newly-qualified doctor is likely to meet and have to begin to cope with before more experienced help arrives. The format of question and answer gives more scope for testing and imparting knowledge than the 'all pervasive' MCQ and we hope that this book will provide a welcome and stimulating change.

We would like to thank Mr Michael Kelly for suggesting that we should write a companion to his own book, Dr John Gillman of John Wright & Sons Ltd for his continual help and encouragement in the preparation of this book, Mrs Maura Mallon for her expert typing of the manuscript and finally our colleagues who have been very tolerant of our questions seeking to clarify various points.

B. T. C.
M. J. H.

# Contents

# How to use this book

The questions are to be found on the right hand page and the answers are placed on the back of the same page. The sections on the various medical specialities are arranged in alphabetical order. Use of the index permits revision of topics that are covered in several sections of the book.

# Accident and Emergency Medicine

1. A shabby middle-aged man is brought into casualty unconscious and smelling of alcohol, having been found in a gutter. What diagnostic pitfall can occur?

2. What are your first actions when an unconscious patient is brought into casualty?

3. How do you treat hysterical overbreathing?

4. What is the treatment of status epilepticus?

5. What important diagnosis can easily be missed in young adults with chest pain?

6. How would you control a violent patient who is restrained only by 4 large policemen?

7. An 85-year-old lady is brought into casualty because of a sudden onset of mental confusion. What diagnosis would you consider?

*Answers overleaf*

1. The main danger is that because the police, ambulancemen and nurses think that the patient is 'dead drunk' you will assume the same. You must make sure that there is no other disorder causing the unconsciousness. Particular pitfalls are missing a head injury, hypoglycaemia in a diabetic, a drug overdose or a post-ictal state.

2. Check that the patient has an adequate airway, is breathing satisfactorily and has a satisfactory pulse and blood pressure. Relevant treatment must be started at once if any vital signs are dangerously abnormal. Only after this can assessment, diagnosis and further treatment take place.

3. If reassurance does not work, consider mild sedation. If this is ineffective, make the patient rebreathe $CO_2$ into a bag.

4. Maintain airway and oxygenation. In severe cases, especially if the fits are not rapidly controlled, paralyse and ventilate the patient. Control fits with diazepam—10 mg i.v.stat. followed by 50–100 mg slowly by i.v. infusion. Continue for 12 hours after last fit. Paraldehyde i.m. or chlormethiazole by i.v. infusion can be used if diazepam is ineffective. Start oral treatment as soon as is practical.
Treat underlying cause and maintain fluid and electrolyte balance.

5. Spontaneous pneumothorax.

6. Chlorpromazine or haloperidol i.m. is usually effective. Paraldehyde is an effective alternative.

7. Any acute illness may precipitate confusion in elderly people. Common causes are myocardial infarction, heart failure, infections (e.g. pneumonia; urinary tract infections; septicaemia), neurological diseases (e.g. cerebrovascular accident; subdural haematoma), shock, dehydration, metabolic problems (e.g. uraemia, hyponatraemia, hypoglycaemia, hyperglycaemia, hypercalcaemia), drugs (especially hypnotics and sedatives). Remember that the cause may be less prominent than the confusional state and that a chronically demented patient may be brought into casualty by relatives or friends as an 'acute confusional state'.

**8.** Outline, in general terms, the treatment of shock.

**9.** How do you manage hypothermia?

**10.** What disorders may produce severe life-threatening upper airways obstruction in adults?

*Answers overleaf*

**8.** The aim of treatment is to restore cardiac output and tissue perfusion rapidly. Therefore:

Give oxygen; check blood gases.

Restore effective circulating volume with blood plasma expander or isotonic saline. Monitor fluid infusion with a central venous pressure line or Swan Ganz catheter which monitors pulmonary artery wedge pressure which reflects left atrial pressure.

Give inotropic agent, e.g. dopamine, which increases blood pressure and renal perfusion.

Give digoxin if the shock is precipitated by or is accompanied by heart failure.

Treat underlying cause.

Controversial aspects of treatment are giving vasodilators in patients with intense vasoconstriction and giving massive doses of corticosteroids in patients with gram-negative septicaemic shock.

**9.** Establish an airway and give oxygen.

Monitor blood gases; give bicarbonate if the patient is grossly acidotic.

Expand blood volume and maintain blood pressure; it is important to avoid 'rewarming shock'.

Monitor serum potassium and ECG because of risk of arrhythmias.

Rewarm mild cases externally but in severe cases consider using dialysis (peritoneal or haemo) to raise the core temperature.

Give antibiotics prophylactically to prevent infection.

**10.** Retropharyngeal abscess

Foreign body in the larynx

Carcinoma of the larynx

Ludwig's angina (submandibular cellulitis with swelling and displacement of the tongue)

All these problems require emergency laryngoscopy and/or tracheostomy.

**11.** You are presented with a woman who states she has been raped. What do you do?

**12.** What signs of death do you look for when called to a body?

**13.** When is a death notifiable to the coroner?

*Answers overleaf*

11. Record the date, the time of the patient's arrival and of the examination and by whom the examination was requested.
    Take a detailed history in private including the patient's own account in her own words.
    Obtain full consent, preferably written, for examination which should be carried out at once.
    Observe and record the patient's behaviour, mood and appearance, including the state of her hair, clothes, etc.
    Perform a general examination for scratches and bruises.
    Examine the perineum in the lithotomy position with particular attention to the state of pubic hair, bleeding and bruising of the vulva, tearing of the hymen and condition of the vagina.
    Take a specimen of pubic hair and make thin smears from the vagina on glass slides using a cotton swab.
    Send relevant clothing for examination for seminal and blood stains.
    Write up the full report at once and keep a copy.

12. Absence of respiration
    Absence of pulse or heart beat
    Fixed dilated pupils
    'Cattle trucking' of blood in retinal vessels.

13. Deaths of unknown or uncertain cause including cases when the patient has been seen only after death.
    Deaths in prison or in police custody.
    Violent or unnatural deaths due to:
        Accident, injury, murder
        Drugs or poisons, including alcohol and therapeutic errors
        Neglect, self-neglect, exposure
        Abortions
        Obscure infant deaths
        Industrial disease
        Pensionable disabilities.
    'Anaesthetic' deaths, i.e. perioperative deaths.

**14.** When is a forced alkaline diuresis indicated?

**15.** What are the possible complications of a tricyclic overdose?

**16.** What acid–base abnormalities are associated with salicylate poisoning?

**17.** How would you manage an iron overdose?

*Answers overleaf*

**14.** A forced alkaline diuresis is rarely indicated. It is of use in severe cases of aspirin overdose (plasma level greater than 450 mg/l) and phenobarbitone overdose (deeply unconscious hypotensive patient with plasma level greater than 550 mmol/l). However, it is never essential in either, but in aspirin overdose it may reduce the plasma salicylate level by half in 8 h and it reduces the coma length by two-thirds in a phenobarbitone overdose. It is a dangerous procedure which should not be undertaken lightly and should be done in an intensive care situation with constant monitoring of fluid balance, cardiac rhythm and serum electrolytes. It is contraindicated in patients with severe cardiac disease or renal failure. An alternative for severe overdosage is haemodialysis. Theoretically, other drugs which may be helped by a forced alkaline diuresis are barbitone, nitrofurantoin, phenylbutazone and probenecid. It is not indicated in overdoses of the other barbiturates because they are not excreted by the kidneys.

**15.** Hypotension
Tremor
Hallucinations, confusion, convulsions
Cardiac dysrhythmias.

**16.** The most usual acid–base disturbance is a respiratory alkalosis, although particularly in children, a metabolic acidosis may be found.

**17.** In this order, you would:
Give desferrioxamine 1–2 g i.m. at once.
Washout the stomach with a mildly alkaline solution (1% sodium bicarbonate) to render iron salts less soluble.
Put 5 g desferrioxamine in 100 ml water into the stomach after the washout.
Set up i.v. infusion for electrolyte and fluid replacement.
Give desferrioxamine 1–2 g i.m. 12 hourly or, in severe cases, give desferrioxamine 15 mg/kg/h i.v. to a maximum of 80 mg/kg/ day.
If patient becomes anuric, consider exchange transfusion.

**18.** Should every overdose receive a stomach washout?

**19.** What is the most sinister complication of paracetamol overdosage and how might you prevent it occurring?

**20.** Where can you get information about the effects and possible treatments of poisoning with drugs, chemicals etc.?

**21.** What is the major problem in morphine or other opiate overdosage and what is its treatment?

**22.** Do you know the incidence of self-poisoning in Britain?

**23.** Does every overdose need a psychiatric assessment?

*Answers overleaf*

**18.** This is controversial. Undoubtedly many overdoses receive unnecessary gastric lavage. In conscious children, many doctors would prefer inducing vomiting mechanically, or better still with syrup of ipecac. However, only 30% of the ingested poison can reliably be removed. If no result (ipecac. takes up to 30 min to work) gastric lavage should proceed. Some would follow a similar plan with conscious adults. It is more usual to washout patients within 4 h of ingestion of the poison and in every case of narcotic, salicylate, tricyclic or iron overdosage. If the patient is unconscious, gastric lavage should follow intubation with a cuffed endotracheal tube and any necessary initial resuscitation procedures. Gastric lavage is contraindicated after corrosive or petroleum product ingestion.

**19.** Hepatic cell necrosis; it may be prevented by administration of acetylcysteine i.v. within 10 h of ingestion.

**20.** Poisons information centres; there are four in the United Kingdom situated in London, Cardiff, Edinburgh and Belfast and they are manned 24 hours a day.

**21.** Respiratory depression; naloxone and, if indicated, mechanical ventilation.

**22.** There are approximately 70,000 admissions for self-poisoning per year in the United Kingdom i.e. 1 in 10 of all emergency admissions.

**23.** This is controversial, in particular because of its medicolegal consequences. In most hospitals, it is standard practice for all overdoses to be assessed by a psychiatrist before discharge. However, this is probably a waste of manpower because most cases can be adequately assessed by the house physician and registrar of the admitting firm. Anyway their opinion will be as good as that of the psychiatric SHO who is frequently given the chore of assessing the overdose. Most overdoses are easy to assess and are the result of impulsive or manipulative behaviour. However, elderly over-doses, however minor their attempt at suicide, are more difficult to assess and always need careful assessment by a psychiatrist.

**24.** How would you manage an adverse reaction to a psychodysleptic drug (e.g. L.S.D.)?

**25.** What are the medical complications of opiate addiction?

**26.** Outline the differences between fresh and salt water drowning?

**27.** Is any treatment possible in cyanide poisoning?

**28.** How would you treat carbon monoxide poisoning?

*Answers overleaf*

**24.** Mild cases can be reassured by 'talking the patient down' but requires continual presence of the therapist and is very time-consuming. It is much more practical in the emergency situation to sedate the patient with diazepam and seek psychiatric advice when the patient has recovered.

**25.** Thrombophlebitis and venous thrombosis.
Infections—septicaemia, infective endocarditis, cellulitis, serum (type B) hepatitis, superficial and deep abscess, septic arthritis, meningitis.
Neurological disorders—amblyopia, transverse myelopathy, peripheral neuropathy.
Myopathy, myoglobinuria, renal failure.

**26.** Fresh water drowning leads to aspiration of hypotonic water, the absorption of which leads to pulmonary surfactant damage, alveolar collapse, hypoxia, haemolysis and hyponatraemia.
Salt water drowning leads to aspiration of hypertonic water which causes pulmonary oedema, hypoxia, dehydration and hypernatraemia.
However, these differences are academic as the main serious effect of either form of drowning is hypoxia leading to metabolic acidosis, hypotension, acute tubular necrosis, acute renal failure and cerebral damage.

**27.** Yes, if started at once. The aim of treatment is to give nitrites (amyl or sodium nitrite) to produce methaemoglobin which competes with cytochrome oxidase for cyanide, cobalt edetate which chelates cyanide, and sodium thiosulphate which converts cyanide to inactive thiocyanate. Vigorous support with ventilation, oxygen and pressor agents are also necessary.

**28.** Ventilation with pure oxygen (hyperbaric oxygen may be necessary for severe cases).
Transfusion with fresh red cells.
Keep patient quiet and calm.

**29.** What are the major clinical problems after paraquat poisoning?

**30.** Summarize the management of paraquat poisoning.

**31.** What is the treatment of severe smoke inhalation?

**32.** How would you manage a patient who has been bitten by what he thinks was a poisonous snake?

*Answers overleaf*

**29.** Pulmonary oedema and haemorrhage leading to progressive pulmonary fibrosis which is the most important cause of death; other problems are hepatic and renal failure; mouth and oesophageal ulceration.

**30.** Gastric lavage if less than 4 h after ingestion.
Leave 250 ml of a 30% suspension of Fullers' Earth and a 5% suspension of magnesium sulphate in the stomach.
Repeat this dose 4-hourly until the faecal specimens are negative (no blue colour produced) on testing with alkaline sodium dithionite.
Consider charcoal haemoperfusion if patient presents less than 8 h after ingestion.

**31.** Administration of oxygen. If irritant gases have been inhaled corticosteroids and appropriate therapy for pulmonary oedema may be necessary.

**32.** Reassurance; admit for observation; immobilize bitten part; obtain description or specimen of snake.
Treat locally with incision of the bite and intermittent suction for 1 h; absorption of venom may be reduced by immediate application of a light tourniquet which does not occlude arterial supply; it should be released every 15 min.
Monitor the following: BP, pulse, respiration rate, ECG, white cell count, serum bicarbonate and creatine phosphokinase, urine output, specific gravity and blood urea.
Observe for local necrosis, abnormal bleeding, ptosis, dysphagia and neuromuscular problems.
If necrosis occurs, excision of slough, antibiotics and skin grafting will be required. Antivenom given early may be helpful.
If systemic envenoming occurs, antivenom should be administered, with adrenaline drawn up in a syringe in case of anaphylaxis.
Treat with oxygen, blood transfusion, fluid and electrolytes i.v. and mechanical ventilation as indicated.

# Cardiovascular Medicine

**33.** What are the classic signs of a deep vein thrombosis?

**34.** What changes in the fundi may be seen in hypertension?

**35.** Do you know any reason why the BP in the legs might be lower than that in the arms?

**36.** List some of the side effects that can occur with methyldopa?

**37.** Why is it dangerous to stop hypotensive therapy with clonidine suddenly?

**38.** What is an anacrotic pulse?

**39.** Do you know the causes of a collapsing pulse?

*Answers overleaf*

**33.** Pain, especially in the calves.
Tenderness over the deep veins.
Oedema and increased girth of the limb.
Warmth and dilated superficial veins over the limb.
Positive Homan's sign (should be elicited with great care).
Fever.
N.B. Significant deep venous thrombosis may be present without any of the above.

**34.** Variation in vessel calibre, increased light reflex (silver wiring) (Grade I).
Arteriovenous nipping (Grade II).
Haemorrhages and soft, fluffy, white (cotton wool) exudates (Grade III).
Papilloedema (Grade IV).

**35.** Coarctation of the aorta.
Atheromatous narrowing of the aorta, iliac or femoral arteries.

**36.** Drug fever, rashes, sedation+, weakness+, headache.
Postural hypotension, oedema.
Nausea, vomiting, constipation, diarrhoea, dry mouth+, 'black' tongue, pancreatitis*.
Jaundice, liver disease*.
Positive Coombs' test+, haemolytic anaemia*, leucopenia*, thrombocytopenia*.
Loss of libido+, impotence+, galactorrhoea, gynaecomastia.

+common        *rare

**37.** Rebound hypertension.

**38.** Prolonged pulse of small amplitude with a notch on the upstroke; characteristic of aortic stenosis; also called 'plateau pulse'.

**39.** Aortic incompetence.
Any condition causing a high output state, e.g. fever, thyrotoxicosis, arteriovenous fistulae (as in Paget's disease of bone, or after trauma), wet beri-beri (thiamine deficiency), $CO_2$ retention, patent ductus arteriosus.

**40.** Where and in what circumstances might you hear a 'pistol shot' with your stethoscope?

**41.** What lesions can cause a pansystolic murmur maximal at the 4th interspace at the left sternal edge?

**42.** How do you diagnose complete heart block at the bed side?

**43.** What is the treatment of paroxysmal supraventricular tachycardia?

**44.** What are the indications for digoxin?

**45.** What percentage of people with rheumatic carditis give a history of rheumatic fever?

*Answers overleaf*

**40.** Over the femoral arteries in aortic incompetence.

**41.** Ventricular septal defect.
Tricuspid incompetence.

**42.** History of blackouts suggesting Stokes Adams attacks (not always present).
Examination revealing a slow regular pulse of about 40/min which does not vary with exercise, irregular 'a' cannon waves in the JVP, and varying first heart sound on auscultation.
Confirmation by ECG.

**43.** Initially carotid sinus massage (one side at a time) but it is difficult to do properly and is unpleasant for the patient.
Verapamil 5 mg i.v. is probably the drug of choice—repeat 5–10 min later; do not give with β-blockers, within 12 h of β-blockers or if there is A–V block.
Practolol 10 mg i.v. can be given as second choice—repeat once after 15 min; do not give within 30 min of verapamil or if the patient is in heart failure.
Synchronized D.C. cardioversion, if drugs have no effect.
Disopyramide may be used as an alternative drug acutely or as maintenance therapy to prevent recurrence.
For a slower conversion to sinus rhythm, digoxin (if no A–V block) or phenytoin (if there is A–V block) may be given.
Digoxin, phenytoin, β-blockers, procainamide, disopyramide or amiodarone may be used to prevent relapse.

**44.** Uncontrolled atrial fibrillation, atrial flutter, paroxysmal atrial tachycardia and heart failure; its use in cardiac failure with sinus rhythm is debatable; it is probably of little value in cor pulmonale.

**45.** About 50%.

**46.** What are the diagnostic criteria for rheumatic fever?

**47.** What are the typical clinical features of aortic stenosis?

**48.** Which valve is most commonly involved in rheumatic carditis?

**49.** What are the causes of mitral incompetence?

**50.** What signs might you see in subacute infective endocarditis?

*Answers overleaf*

**46.** Jones criteria (revised):
Major: carditis, polyarthritis, Sydenham's chorea, subcutaneous nodules, erythema marginatum.
Minor: previous rheumatic fever or carditis, arthralgia, fever, raised ESR and leucocytosis, prolonged P–R interval on ECG.
Two major, one minor, and evidence of previous streptococcal infection (ASO titres raised; positive culture; scarlet fever) or one major, two minor and evidence of previous streptococcal infection makes the diagnosis very likely.

**47.** Symptoms: dyspnoea, angina, blackouts (syncopal attacks).
Signs: anacrotic pulse, narrow pulse pressure, signs of left ventricular hypertrophy, ejection systolic murmur maximal at the second right interspace radiating to the carotids with an ejection click at the start of the murmur (in young people) and often associated with a systolic thrill.

**48.** Mitral valve.

**49.** Rheumatic heart disease
Dilated left ventricle
Papillary muscle dysfunction after myocardial infarct or ischaemia
Prolapsed cusp (floppy valve)
After mitral valvotomy for mitral stenosis
Bacterial endocarditis
Congenital
Endocardial cushion defect.

**50.** Fever
Pallor
Cafe-au-lait complexion (late)
Petechiae
Splinter haemorrhages
Osler's nodes on fingers and toes
Janeway lesions on palms and soles
Clubbing (mild in long standing cases)
Splenomegaly
Flame-shaped haemorrhages and Roth spots on fundi
Microscopic haematuria
Evidence of valvular or structural heart disease, or coarctation of aorta
Evidence of embolic damage, e.g. CVA.

**51.** How do you prevent subacute bacterial endocarditis?

**52.** List the causes of hypertension secondary to some recognizable underlying factor.

**53.** What should you do if you suspect an arterial embolus in a leg, and what is the treatment of choice?

*Answers overleaf*

**51.** Antibiotic cover for any procedure, however minor, especially involving mouth, teeth, pharynx, and upper respiratory tract; but do not forget gastrointestinal, gynaecological and urological procedures.

**52.** Renal disease (can be seen in virtually all types), e.g.:
Acute and chronic glomerulonephritis
Diabetic nephropathy
Chronic pyelonephritis
Polycystic disease
Unilateral renal ischaemia (e.g. renal artery stenosis)
Obstructive uropathy.

Endocrine disease:
Cushing's syndrome
Corticosteroid or ACTH therapy
Primary aldosteronism (Conn's syndrome)
Phaeochromocytoma.

Other disease:
Coarctation of the aorta
Toxaemia of pregnancy
Acute onset raised intracranial pressure, e.g. after subarachnoid haemorrhage
Interaction of MAO inhibitors (given for depression) with foods containing tyramine, e.g. cheese, beans
Oestrogen/progestogen contraceptive pill.

**53.** Keep the patient warm but the affected limb cool and at rest
Give analgesics
Heparin 5000 units i.v. followed by Heparin infusion
Call a surgeon
Look for a source for the embolus (aortic aneurysm, myocardial infarction, atrial fibrillation, prosthetic heart valve, SBE) and initiate treatment where appropriate.
Embolectomy is the treatment of choice and should be performed within 8 h of the embolus; minor embolism, distal embolism, irreversible ischaemia, or delay after 8 h requires continued medical therapy with anticoagulants. Amputation may be necessary for severe pain or gangrene.
Long-term anticoagulation may be necessary to prevent recurrence.
There seems to be no place for vasodilator drugs.

**54.** What are Kerley B lines?

**55.** What are the side effects of digoxin?

**56.** What is a silent myocardial infarct?

**57.** What are the clinical features of a massive pulmonary embolus?

*Answers overleaf*

**54.** Small transverse lines seen in the peripheries of the lung fields on chest X-rays of patients with pulmonary oedema; they are caused by fluid in the interlobular septa.

**55.** Anorexia
Nausea, vomiting
Headache
Fatigue
Dreams, restlessness, agitation
Visual blurring and xanthopsia (yellow vision)
Bradycardia (often with A–V conduction defects)
Arrhythymias, especially ventricular ectopics with coupling (more likely if patient is hypokalaemic)
Gynaecomastia.

**56.** A painless infarct; they are probably quite common in that patients are often seen with features of an old infarct on ECG but no associated history; they are more common in diabetics and the elderly; they may present with the complications of myocardial infarction

**57.** Symptoms: dyspnoea (most important)
crushing central chest pain
fainting.

Signs: cyanosis, tachycardia, hypotension, cold peripheries
signs of acute right ventricular strain: JVP raised, right ventricular (parasternal) heave, loud pulmonary second sound, triple (gallop) rhythm
pulmonary systolic murmur (very rare).

**58.** What are the risk factors for a deep vein thrombosis?

**59.** What is the usual cause of early death after a myocardial infarct?

**60.** Why do you treat postmyocardial infarct ventricular ectopics, when are they significant and how do you treat them?

**61.** Approximately how many deaths from ischaemic heart disease occur in England and Wales per annum?

**62.** How do you treat acute left ventricular failure?

*Answers overleaf*

**58.** Immobilization
Cardiac failure
Tight belts, garters, etc.
Surgery, especially on pelvis
Pregnancy
Dehydration
Myocardial infarction
Pelvic tumours
Ulcerative colitis
Diseases associated with hyperviscosity (e.g. polycythaemia, multiple myeloma)
Oestrogen-containing 'pill' (especially associated with smoking)
Carcinoma.

**59.** Ventricular fibrillation.

**60.** Because of the risk of their precipitating ventricular tachycardia and fibrillation.
Significant ectopics occur on top of the preceding T waves (R on T phenomenon), at more than 5 per min, or in runs.
The best treatment is lignocaine by i.v. infusion 1–4 mg/min—mexiletine or disopyramide may be used intravenously as alternatives as well as orally for maintenance therapy long term.

**61.** 110000.

**62.** Initially:
Keep patient sitting up
High concentration of oxygen and morphine 10 mg i.v. (provided the patient does not have obstructive airways disease)
A loop diuretic i.v., e.g. frusemide 40 mg
Digitalize if uncontrolled atrial fibrillation.
If poor response:
Repeat i.v. diuretic
Digitalize (if not done already)
Consider a vasodilator drug.
In extreme cases:
Ventilation.

**63.** In which leads are the ECG changes of acute lateral myocardial infarction seen?

**64.** What conditions can present as angina pectoris?

**65.** In what ways can ischaemic heart disease present?

**66.** What are the characteristics of pulsus alternans and pulsus paradoxus?

**67.** What is a cannon wave and in what circumstances is it found?

*Answers overleaf*

**63.** Leads I, AVL and $V_{4-6}$.

**64.** Atheroma
Aortic stenosis
Anaemia
Hypothyroidism
Hyperlipidaemia
Diabetes mellitus
Paroxysmal tachycardia
Syphilis
Polyarteritis nodosa

**65.** Angina pectoris
Myocardial infarction
Sudden death
Cardiac failure
Arrythmias
Conduction defects

**66.** Pulsus alternans is regular alternation of pulse pressure despite a regular rhythm, and is indicative of left ventricular decompensation.
Pulsus paradoxus is an accentuation of the normal reduction in pulse pressure occurring in inspiration. It is typically present in severe airways obstruction, cardiac tamponade, and constrictive pericarditis.

**67.** It is a large jugular venous 'a' wave produced by contractions of the right atrium against a closed tricuspid valve, such as in complete heart block.

**68.** Give some examples of added sounds in cardiac auscultation and to what are they due?

**69.** When is the diaphragm and when is the bell of a stethoscope used? Give examples.

**70.** What are the causes of atrial fibrillation?

**71.** Outline a regimen for the oral digitalization of a patient with atrial fibrillation with a ventricular rate of 130 per min, using digoxin.

*Answers overleaf*

**68.** 3rd heart sound—rapid filling of the ventricles in first part of diastole, normal in children but indicative of LV decompensation in patients over 40.

4th heart sound—filling of ventricles during later part of diastole due to atrial contraction and diminished ventricular compliance.

Opening snap—in early diastole due to rapid opening of stenosed mitral valve.

Ejection click—in early systole due to rapid opening of stenosed aortic (or pulmonary) valve.

Mid systolic click—often in association with late systolic murmur due to prolapse of the posterior leaflet of mitral valve in some cases of mitral incompetence.

**69.** Diaphragm—high pitched sounds—systolic murmurs, early diastolic murmur of aortic incompetence, opening snap, ejection click.

Bell—low pitched sounds—mid-diastolic murmur of mitral stenosis, 3rd and 4th heart sounds.

**70.** Ischaemic heart disease
Mitral valve disease
Thyrotoxicosis
Hypertension
Fever
Pulmonary embolus
Cardiomyopathies
Post thoracotomy
'Lone' fibrillation.

**71.** 0·5–1·5 mg digoxin orally (depending on weight) followed by 0·25 mg three times daily until digitalized. Thereafter maintenance therapy of 0·25 once or twice daily is usually sufficient. If the clinical condition of the patient is satisfactory the loading dose can be omitted and digitalization using a maintenance dosage can be expected after 5 days. The elderly are sensitive to digoxin and may require a much reduced maintenance dose, even as low as 0·0625 mg daily. In renal failure the dose of digoxin should also be reduced.

**72.**   List the recognized risk factors for ischaemic heart disease.

**73.**   A man presents to the casualty department with a history of sudden onset of severe central chest pain. What is the differential diagnosis?

**74.**   What investigations would you perform to confirm myocardial injury in a patient admitted to hospital with a suspected diagnosis of myocardial infarction?

**75.**   What are the radiographic features on a PA chest X-ray of pulmonary embolism and/or infarction?

**76.**   What are the symptoms of uncomplicated hypertension?

*Answers overleaf*

**72.** Cigarette smoking
Hypertension
Hyperlipidaemia
Diabetes mellitus
Family history
Obesity (but only in its association with hypertension).

**73.** Myocardial infarction
Myocardial ischaemia without infarction
Pericarditis
Gastro-oesophageal reflux, oesophagitis or oesophageal spasm
Non-specific chest wall pain (e.g. left submammary pain syndrome)
Anxiety/neurosis
Pulmonary embolus
Dissection of aorta
Bornholm disease (epidemic myalgia due to Coxsackie B virus)
Dorsal spinal lesions
Tietze's syndrome (costochondritis of upper costochondral cartilages).

**74.** Neutrophil count
ESR
Cardiac enzymes—creatinine phosphokinase
aspartate aminotransferase (SGOT)
lactate dehydrogenase or its isoenzymes
Electrocardiogram.

**75.** Pulmonary embolus:
abrupt cut off of major pulmonary vessel.
area of increased radiolucency.
Pulmonary infarction:
area of opacity typically wedge-shaped with base abutting to pleura.
linear opacity (plate atelectasis)
pleural effusion
raised hemidiaphragm.
N.B. The chest X-ray may be normal.

**76.** Usually none, although complaints of headaches, dizziness, palpitation and easy fatigability are often attributed to hypertension.

**77.** Outline the investigations you would perform in a 35-year-old man in whom hypertension was the only abnormality discovered at an insurance medical examination.

**78.** What are the complications of hypertension?

**79.** List the most important drugs or groups of drugs currently used in the treatment of hypertension.

**80.** Name the organisms most commonly found in infective endocarditis.

**81.** To what signs do Austin Flint, Graham Steell and Osler refer? In what conditions are they found?

*Answers overleaf*

**77.** Urinalysis for protein, blood and glucose; urine microscopy and culture.
Blood urea, creatinine, electrolytes, glucose.
Full blood count.
Chest X-ray.
Electrocardiogram.
Further investigations would be indicated if a secondary cause is suggested by above or arterial pressure fails to come under control after initial therapy.

**78.** Cardiac — left ventricular hypertrophy and failure
atrial fibrillation
increased risk of ischaemic heart disease.
Cerebral — cerebral ischaemia
cerebral haemorrhage
hypertensive encephalopathy.
Renal — renal failure
Eyes — hypertensive retinopathy.

**79.** Diuretics, particularly the thiazides
Beta-blocking drugs
Centrally acting anti-adrenergic drugs, e.g. methyldopa
Vasodilators e.g. prazosin, hydralazine
Angiotensin-converting enzyme inhibitors, e.g. captopril, saralsin
Adrenergic neurone blocking drugs, e.g. reserpine and guanethidine.
Some patients with long-standing hypertension are still taking these drugs, but they should only be used in new patients if other regimens fail.

**80.** *Streptococcus viridans, Streptococcus faecalis, Staphylococcus aureus, Coxiella burnetii,* fungi.

**81.** Austin Flint — low pitched rumbling mid-diastolic murmur due to displacement of the anterior leaflet of mitral valve in patients with aortic incompetence.
Graham Steell — high pitched diastolic murmur of pulmonary incompetence in severe pulmonary hypertension due to mitral stenosis.
Osler — subcutaneous tender erythematous papules on the pulp of fingers and toes in infective endocarditis, so-called Osler's nodes.

**82.** Compare and contrast the auscultatory features of mitral stenosis and aortic incompetence.

**83.** What are the physical signs of tricuspid incompetence?

**84.** Name 3 investigations which may be useful in diagnosis of deep venous thrombosis.

**85.** What is 'maladie de Roger'?

**86.** Describe the ECG changes which may occur with uncomplicated acute myocardial infarction.

*Answers overleaf*

**82.** Mitral stenosis — accentuation of 1st heart sound
opening snap
low pitched, rumbling mid-diastolic murmur
best heard at the apex; with presystolic
accentuation if the patient is in sinus
rhythm.

Aortic incompetence — high pitched, blowing, decrescendo early
diastolic murmur best heard in 3rd
intercostal space at the left sternal
border.
In addition, other murmurs are sometimes
heard e.g. the Austin Flint murmur—a soft
low pitched rumbling mid diastolic
murmur produced by displacement of the
mitral valve by regurgitant stream; a
systolic ejection murmur due to increased
blood flow.

**83.** Raised jugular venous pressure, strongly pulsatile due to prominent 'v'
waves; hepatomegaly with systolic pulsation of liver; pansystolic
murmur at lower left sternal border increased during inspiration.

**84.** Ultrasound (Doppler) flow technique
Radiolabelled ($1^{131}$) fibrinogen uptake
Contrast venography (phlebography).

**85.** A small ventricular septal defect.

**86.** T wave inversion
ST elevation
Q waves.

87. A man of 45 years presents with chest pain and is found to have a pericardial friction rub. Give the differential diagnosis.

88. List some conditions for which echocardiography is useful in diagnosis.

89. What abnormalities comprise Fallot's tetralogy?

90. Give the drug treatment which is available for angina pectoris.

91. What is the incidence of congenital cardiac abnormalities?

92. What is the cause of the murmur in ostium secundum (common) type of atrial septal defect?

*Answers overleaf*

**87.** Pericarditis due to: viral infection
myocardial infarction
uraemia
infiltrating carcinoma
tuberculosis
collagen vascular disease, e.g. rheumatoid arthritis, SLE
post-myocardial infarction (Dressler's) syndrome
post-pericardiotomy
myxoedema
trauma.

**88.** Pericardial effusion
Mitral valve disease
Atrial myxoma
Infective endocarditis
Cardiomyopathy.

**89.** Pulmonary stenosis
Ventricular septal defect
Overriding of the aorta
Right ventricular hypertrophy.

**90.** Nitrates:
short-acting—glyceryl trinitrate (sublingual or paste)
long-acting—e.g. pentaerythritol tetranitrate (oral), isosorbide dinitrate (oral)
β-blockers—e.g. propranolol, atenolol
Calcium antagonists—e.g. nifedipine.

**91.** 1% of live births.

**92.** Increased flow across the pulmonary valve during systole.

**93.** What is the Wenkebach phenomenon?

**94.** Outline the principles of management of a cardiac arrest.

*Answers overleaf*

**93.** Second-degree heart block with a progressive increase in PR interval until a ventricular beat is dropped completely (also called Mobitz type 1 heart block).

**94.** Establish an airway. Mouth-to-mouth resuscitation may be necessary and is facilitated by a Brook airway. If the equipment is available, endotracheal intubation and ventilation with oxygen is the method of choice.

Perform cardiac massage. Before performing above, an immediate blow to the precordium is sometimes successful. 'Blind' defibrillation without waiting for a rhythm diagnosis is often worthwhile.

Establish intravenous access and give 100 mM (100 ml of 8·4%) sodium bicarbonate. Repeat after 10 min, but thereafter arterial blood gases should be checked. The intravenous line should be kept open with 5% dextrose.

Obtain electrocardiographic monitoring, often available via the paddles of the defibrillator, and make a rhythm diagnosis.

Treat the rhythm abnormality
Asystole—1 ml of 1 in 1000 adrenaline intravenously or, if no satisfactory venous access, by the intracardiac route. 10 ml 10% calcium gluconate intravenously (but not via the same infusion as the sodium bicarbonate). If no success, consider transvenous or direct intracardiac pacing.

Ventricular fibrillation—Defibrillation with 100 joules increasing to the maximum, usually 400 joules, if necessary, followed by lignocaine infusion (1–4 mg/min). Failure or relapse should be treated by further defibrillation and the bolus administration of 100 mg lignocaine.

# Endocrinology and Diabetes

**95.**  Do you know the incidence of diabetes mellitus in Great Britain?

**96.**  What is a potential diabetic?

**97.**  List the types of coma seen in diabetics.

**98.**  How would you treat hypoglycaemia?

**99.**  Outline the usual insulin regimes used in the treatment of diabetes mellitus.

*Answers overleaf*

**95.** About 1% of the population—80% of diabetics are of maturity onset type.

**96.** A person who is at risk of developing diabetes because of a strong family history or a poor obstetric history (i.e. overweight babies, unexplained fetal deaths).

**97.** Ketoacidosis
Hypoglycaemia
Non-ketotic hyperosmolar coma
Lactic acidosis
N.B. Do not forget that unrelated disorders may cause coma in diabetic patients.

**98.** If at all possible, check blood sugar on blood sugar dipsticks (e.g. Dextrostix) and take a venous sample for accurate blood sugar estimation; ignore any urinalysis results. If the patient is conscious enough to swallow and cough, give glucose 10–20 g by mouth; if the patient is unconscious, give dextrose 50% 50 ml i.v. or glucagon 1 mg i.m. (if poor veins). Beware recurring hypoglycaemia if the patient has taken long-acting insulin or sulphonylurea (especially chlorpropamide).

**99.** There are many different regimes but two basic ones are commonly used.
Twice-daily soluble and isophane insulin, used for the great majority of diabetics, is flexible and provides good control. Soluble insulin—onset 15 min, peak 3–5 h, duration 6–8 h; isophane (NPH) insulin—onset 2 h, peak 5–12 h, duration 16–28 h.
Once-daily insulin, usually lente—used for patients who cannot or will not take two injections a day, provided they do not rapidly become ketoacidotic without insulin. Control is often suboptimal but is particularly useful in elderly diabetics. However, change to twice daily regime is often necessary, especially if the total dose exceeds 60 units/day. Other problems include midmorning glycosuria, which may benefit from the addition of neutral soluble insulin, with the morning lente, and nocturnal hypoglycaemia. Lente insulin (insulin zinc suspension [mixed]) contains 30% semilente and 70% ultralente; onset 3 h, peak 6–14 h, duration 22–30 h.

**100.** What features may be seen in diabetic retinopathy?

**101.** What is the commonest cause of death among diabetics?

**102.** What drugs other than insulin are used for treating diabetes mellitus?

**103.** How would you monitor treatment in diabetics?

*Answers overleaf*

**100.** Retinal: microaneurysms, haemorrhages (blot and dot), exudates (hard, waxy but occasionally soft, cotton wool), enlargement and irregularity of veins ('string of sausages'), new vessel formation, detachment.

Preretinal: vitreous haze, vitreous haemorrhage, new vessel formation, fibrosis, vitreous detachment.

Preretinal abnormalities, retinal detachment, new vessel formation and extreme venous irregularity are serious and require expert ophthalmological assessment.

**101.** Ischaemic heart disease—50%; other common causes of death are cerebrovascular disease (12%), renal failure (10%), cancer (10%), infections (6%). Diabetic coma only accounts for 1% of deaths.

**102.** Two groups:

Sulphonylureas—first choice. Act by stimulating insulin production from islet cells, therefore can cause hypoglycaemia. Many different types with different lengths of action, metabolism, routes of excretion and price. Beware of long-acting drugs, e.g. chlorpropamide, gliclazide in the elderly and take care in patients with renal or hepatic failure. In renal failure, choose drug fully metabolized in the liver to inactive metabolites, e.g. tolbutamide; in hepatic failure, choose drug which is not metabolized and is excreted by the kidneys, e.g. chlorpropamide.

Biguanides—indicated for obese patients who cannot lose weight (biguanides have an appetite-suppressant effect) and for use in conjunction with sulphonylureas. They act by increasing peripheral utilization of glucose. Metformin is the drug of choice, although it can cause lactic acidosis.

**103.** Traditional monitoring by urine testing (Clinitest or Diastix) is often misleading and random blood sugars in the clinic are frequently useless. There have been two advances:

Home monitoring of capillary blood sugar by the patient using blood sugar dipsticks which can be read by eye or by commercially available reflectance meters.

Glycosylated haemoglobin measurement. This gives an integrated index of blood sugar levels over the previous 6–8 weeks.

**104.** What types of foot ulcer are seen in diabetics?

**105.** Is there any evidence that good control leads to fewer diabetic complications?

**106.** Are there any advantages in using highly purified (monocomponent) insulins?

**107.** What are the causes of secondary diabetes mellitus?

**108.** Is a glucose tolerance test mandatory in the diagnosis of diabetes mellitus?

*Answers overleaf*

**104.** Ischaemic
Neuropathic
Septic
Mixed.

**105.** The only hard evidence is provided by pregnant diabetics who deliver normal babies when their blood sugar is closely controlled throughout the pregnancy. There is less convincing evidence that retinopathy is associated with poor control. However, it is an article of faith for diabetics and diabetologists that good control reduces the risk of long-term complications.

**106.** Yes; no lipoatrophy, no local or generalized allergic reactions, less chance of insulin antibodies or resistance, lower total insulin dosage, and possibly a favourable effect on long-term complications.

**107.** Common — Acute pancreatitis (usually temporary)
Carcinoma of the pancreas
Chronic pancreatitis
Pancreatectomy (total or subtotal)
Steroid therapy
Thiazide therapy
Cirrhosis of the liver

Rare — Cushing's syndrome
Acromegaly
Haemochromatosis
Phaeochromocytoma
Severe burns (usually temporary)
Glucagonoma (very rare)

**108.** No, the great majority of diabetics are diagnosed by having a random blood sugar of greater than 11 mmol/l. A random blood sugar of less than 8 mmol/l excludes the diagnosis. A random blood sugar of 8–11 mmol/l is equivocal and a 50 g glucose tolerance test is necessary to establish the diagnosis.

N.B. The presence or absence of glycosuria is irrelevant in the diagnosis, although glycosuria often alerts the doctor to the presence of diabetes in a patient.

**109.** What is Graves' disease?

**110.** List the different methods of treating thyrotoxicosis.

**111.** Outline the advantages and disadvantages of drug treatment of thyrotoxicosis.

**112.** How can hyperthyroidism present in the elderly?

**113.** Why do you have to be particularly careful when starting thyroxine in patients with hypothyroidism, especially if they are elderly?

*Answers overleaf*

**109.** It is diffuse hyperplasia of the thyroid gland, leading to thyrotoxicosis. The stimulus to hyperplasia seems to be a thyroid-stimulating immunoglobulin. It is much more common in females, F : M = 8 : 1, and is the only type of thyroid disease associated with exophthalmos, pretibial myxoedema and acropachy.

**110.** Three options:
Antithyroid drugs, e.g. carbimazole
Partial thyroidectomy
Radioiodine.

**111.** Advantages of drugs (e.g. carbimazole)—convenience; avoidance of operation; do not harm fetus in conventional dosage; any hypothyroidism produced is rapidly reversed by reducing dose or stopping drug.

Disadvantages of drugs: long-term treatment (12–18 months); no reduction in gland size (therefore contraindicated in retrosternal goitre); relapse possible after stopping drug and relapse may be resistant to further drug therapy; side effects especially aplastic anaemia and agranulocytosis.

**112.** In the elderly, thyrotoxicosis may present with thyrotoxic heart disease rather than the more familiar symptoms and signs of thyrotoxicosis. Thyrotoxicosis causes tachycardia, vasodilatation and increased cardiac output which may lead eventually to heart failure, most usually associated with atrial fibrillation.

N.B. Thyrotoxicosis can precipitate heart failure from other causes, e.g. ischaemic heart disease.

**113.** Too vigorous institution of thyroxine therapy can lead to clinically overt ischaemic heart disease, because hypothyroidism is associated with an increased incidence of atheroma.

**114.** What is thyroid acropachy?

**115.** What types of neoplasia occur in the thyroid gland?

**116.** What are the clinical and biochemical features of Addison's disease?

**117.** How would you investigate a suspected case of Cushing's syndrome?

*Answers overleaf*

**114.** Clubbing and distal interphalangeal joint arthropathy in patients with Graves' disease.

**115.** Adenoma ('hot' or 'cold' nodules).
Carcinomas derived from follicular epithelium—papillary (commonest), follicular, anaplastic (least common).
Carcinoma derived from parafollicular cells—medullary carcinoma (very rare).
Lymphoma.

**116.** Symptoms: Insidious onset of lethargy, tiredness, postural hypotension, anorexia, nausea, vomiting, diarrhoea or constipation.
Signs: Hypotension, pigmentation (especially in exposed areas and areas subjected to friction) and, in severe cases, dehydration, stupor, coma (partly related to spontaneous hypoglycaemia) and pyrexia.
Biochemistry—low serum sodium, raised serum potassium and blood urea. In mild cases electrolytes and urea may be normal. A low blood sugar may be seen.

**117.** Confirmation of the diagnosis:
Serum cortisol at 8 a.m. and midnight—elevated midnight cortisol and loss of diurnal variation are characteristic of the disorder.
24-hour urine hydroxycorticosteroids and 17 ketogenic steroids —elevated.
Low-dose dexamethasone suppression test (2 mg/day for 2 days)— failure to suppress urinary hydroxycorticosteroid production confirms diagnosis.
Detection of cause:
Serum ACTH—high in adrenal hyperplasia due to excess pituitary production or in ectopic production (usually oat cell bronchial carcinoma).
High-dose dexamethasone suppression test (8 mg/day for 2 days). Suppression of urinary hydroxycorticosteroid production suggests adrenal hyperplasia due to excess pituitary ACTH; failure to suppress suggests adrenal adenoma or carcinoma, or ectopic ACTH source.
Production of 17 ketogenic steroids—much higher in adrenal carcinoma than adenoma.
Search for tumour—adrenal or ectopic.

**118.** Are the terms Cushing's disease and Cushing's syndrome interchangeable?

**119.** What other diseases may be associated with idiopathic Addison's disease?

**120.** How would you establish the diagnosis of adrenal insufficiency?

**121.** Anorexia nervosa is usually listed in the differential diagnosis of panhypopituitarism. Are they easily confused?

**122.** What are the causes of diabetes insipidus?

**123.** How do you treat hypopituitarism?

*Answers overleaf*

**118.** Strictly no; Cushing's disease is specifically adrenal cortical hyperfunction as a result of excess pituitary ACTH. Cushing's syndrome is chronic glucocorticoid excess from any cause.

**119.** Hashimoto's thyroiditis, diabetes mellitus, idiopathic hypoparathyroidism, pernicious anaemia, primary ovarian failure.

**120.** By performing an ACTH stimulation test; there are various variations and modifications but the most accurate is the 'long synacthen test' in which cortisol response to an 8-h ACTH infusion is measured. The simplest screening test is the 'short synacthen test' in which ACTH 25 units is given i.m. and plasma cortisol levels are measured before and at 30 and 60 min after the ACTH. It can occasionally give false positive results.

**121.** In practice—no. While both cause amenorrhoea, there are striking clinical differences. The patient with panhypopituitarism is well nourished and mentally slow or stuporose, whereas the anorexic is emaciated but is very active mentally and physically.

**122.** Cranial causes: hypothalamic and pituitary disease, e.g. tumour (usually metastases), haemorrhage, abscess, meningitis, TB, syphilis, head injury, pituitary surgery, idiopathic.
Nephrogenic: inherited, acquired.

**123.** Treat ACTH deficiency—cortisone acetate (or equivalent)—fludrocortisone is not usually needed as most patients can produce enough aldosterone from their adrenal cortex.

Treat TSH deficiency—thyroxine—never start until patient is established on cortisone because of risk of precipitating Addisonian crisis.

Treat sex hormone deficiency as required—oestrogens, progesterone, androgens.

Treat gonadotrophin deficiency if fertility required—human HCG.

Treat GH deficiency in children—human GH.

**124.** What types of hyperparathyroidism do you know?

**125.** What are the commoner endocrine syndromes resulting from ectopic hormone production by bronchial carcinoma?

**126.** What is Sheehan's syndrome?

**127.** What are the important complications of undescended testes?

**128.** What drugs can cause gynaecomastia?

**129.** List some of the medical complications of the combined oestrogen-progestogen contraceptive pill.

**130.** What do you suspect when a patient, in whom previous bilateral adrenalectomy has been performed for Cushing's disease, complains of increasing skin and mucosal pigmentation?

*Answers overleaf*

**124.** Primary—hyperplasia, adenoma, carcinoma of parathyroid glands.

Secondary—hyperplasia of the parathyroids as a result of hypocalcaemia caused by osteomalacia, malabsorption, chronic renal failure.

Tertiary—persisting hyperplasia of the parathyroid glands after removal of the stimulus to secondary hyperparathyroidism.

**125.** Commoner syndromes are:

From oat-cell carcinoma
Cushing's syndrome due to ACTH production
Inappropriate ADH production
Pigmentation due to MSH production

From squamous cell carcinoma
Hypercalcaemia due to parathormone production or production of other calcium mobilizing substances.

**126.** Hypopituitarism following infarction of the anterior pituitary, due to hypotension resulting from ante- or post-partum haemorrhage.

**127.** Impaired or absent spermatogenesis; malignant change.

**128.** Oestrogens, spironolactone, cimetidine, digoxin, reserpine, methyldopa, isoniazid.

**129.** Hypertension, cerebrovascular accident, venous thromboembolism, gallstones, cholestasis, hepatic adenoma. The risk of vascular complications is greatly increased by concurrent smoking, diabetes mellitus, hyperlipidaemia, hypertension and obesity.

**130.** Nelson's syndrome due to an ACTH-secreting pituitary tumour occurring in 10–15% patients who· have undergone bilateral adrenalectomy for Cushing's disease. The increased pigmentation is due to the melanocyte-stimulating activity of ACTH.

**131.** What is the management of a patient with a solitary thyroid nodule?

**132.** What are the causes of hirsutism in women?

**133.** What is the treatment of hirsutism?

**134.** What are the causes of the syndrome of inappropriate secretion of ADH (SIADH).

*Answers overleaf*

**131.** Establish its functional activity by a radioisotope scan. If there is uptake of the isotope then the nodule is 'hot' and can be left. If it is a 'cold' nodule, i.e. there is reduced or absent uptake of isotope, it should be explored because it may be malignant.

**132.** Organic—often accompanied by other signs of virilization, and include
> congenital adrenal hyperplasia
> ovarian tumours
> adrenal tumours
> and sometimes as a major feature of Cushing's syndrome.

Dysfunctional
> with no well-defined organic cause, but is associated with increased androgen levels.

Idiopathic
> with all androgen levels being normal.

**133.** Organic: treat underlying cause
> Remove ovarian or adrenal tumour
> Suppress with dexamethasone for congenital adrenal hyperplasia.

Dysfunctional
> Treat symptomatically with cyproterone acetate.
> Sometimes the combined contraceptive pill (for ovarian origin) or dexamethasone (for adrenal origin) is used.

Idiopathic
> Bleaching, wax removal or electrolysis. These non-specific methods may be used for all types of hirsutism.

**134.** Oat-cell carcinoma of lung
Carcinoma of pancreas
Tuberculosis
Lung abscess
Pneumonia
Skull fracture
Subdural haematoma
Subarachnoid haemorrhage
Meningitis/encephalitis
Hypothyroidism
Drugs including chlorpropramide, carbamazepine, thiazides, tricyclic antidepressants.

**135.** What would lead you to suspect SIADH?

**136.** What would be the management of SIADH in a patient with an oat-cell carcinoma of the bronchus and a serum sodium of 120 mmol/l?

**137.** Outline the management of goitre.

**138.** What is subclinical or compensated hypothyroidism?

*Anwers overleaf*

**135.** Low serum sodium, i.e. below 130 mmol/l
Urine osmolality $> 300$ mosm/kg
Plasma osmolality $< 275$ mosm/kg
Normal blood urea and creatinine.

**136.** Water restriction 500–1000 ml/day for mild to moderate symptoms of water intoxication.
Demethylchlortetracycline 1200 mg/day is sometimes used.
Severe water intoxication with coma necessitates the use of intravenous hypertonic saline which will increase the serum sodium enough to save the patient's life. However the effect is temporary and allows other treatment to work.
Removal or destruction of the tumour, if at all possible.

**137.** Assess state of thyroid function.
Determine cause— country of origin
dietary history
family history
drug history
thyroid autoantibodies
exclude cancer by thyroid scan.
If non-cancerous, consider surgery for local compression or possibly for cosmetic reasons.
Thyroxine is worth trying (200–300 $\mu$g/day for 6 months).
Reassurance.

**138.** A biochemical finding in which levels of $T_4$ and $T_3$ are normal but a raised TSH suggests the thyroid gland is failing.

**139.** What are the clinical features seen in panhypopituitarism due to a pituitary tumour?

**140.** How would you manage a boy of 14 years with gynaecomastia?

**141.** List the clinical features of acromegaly.

**142.** What investigations would you perform to confirm a suspected diagnosis of acromegaly?

*Answers overleaf*

**139.** The adult patient is usually pale without axillary or pubic hair, has fine wrinkling of the face and poor muscle development.

Specific features due to deficiencies of anterior pituitary hormones including
   thyrotrophin deficiency
   ACTH deficiency
   gonadotrophin deficiency
   growth hormone deficiency
   prolactin deficiency.

Visual disorders—normally visual field defects including, classically, bitemporal hemianopia.

Enlargement of the sella turcica which may be picked up at routine skull X-ray.

**140.** Reassurance. Transient gynaecomastia around puberty is extremely common and in the presence of otherwise normal physical examination, no investigations are indicated. A drug cause should be excluded.

**141.** Thick greasy skin
Prognathism
Broad bulbous nose
Large tongue
Deepening of voice
Broad hands and feet leading to increase in size of rings and footwear
Hypertension
Cardiomegaly
Osteoarthritis
Muscle hypertrophy
Hypercalcaemia
Diabetes mellitus
Signs of expanding lesion in pituitary fossa.

**142.** Measurement of plasma growth hormone during a glucose tolerance test—failure of the normal GH suppression during hyperglycaemia suggests acromegaly; heel pad measurements (normally below 25 mm on lateral radiographs). Other investigations looking for expanding pituitary fossa lesions include pituitary radiology and visual field plotting.

**143.** Categorize the different patterns of diabetic neuropathy.

**144.** List some causes of hyperprolactinaemia.

**145.** What conditions cause thirst and polyuria?

**146.** What is the mode of action of carbimazole?

**147.** Why should a patient be followed up closely after having had thyrotoxicosis successfully treated with $^{131}I$?

**148.** What are the causes of tetany?

*Answers overleaf*

**143.** Peripheral neuropathy
Mononeuropathy including mononeuritis multiplex
Acute painful neuropathy
Diabetic amyotrophy
Autonomic neuropathy.

**144.** Prolactin secreting pituitary microadenomas
Hypothalamic disorders
Hypothyroidism
Renal failure
Ectopic production by malignant tumours
Drugs—dopamine receptor blocking agents, e.g.
phenothiazines, metoclopramide; dopamine depleting agents, e.g.
reserpine, methyldopa, oestrogens, TRH, cimetidine, mono-
amine oxidase inhibitors.

**145.** Diabetes mellitus
Diabetes insipidus
Nephrogenic diabetes insipidus
Hypokalaemia
Hypercalcaemia
Chronic renal failure
Drugs e.g. chlorpromazine, clonidine, lithium, demethylchlor-
tetracycline, diuretics.

**146.** Carbimazole works in two ways:

As an antithyroid drug by blocking the incorporation of iodine
into organic precursors of thyroid hormone.

By reducing the level of thyroid stimulating immunoglobulin in
Graves' disease.

**147.** Because of the risk of hypothyroidism.

**148.** Hypocalcaemia
Hypomagnesaemia
Alkalosis.

**149.** You are called to see a hysterical hyperventilating patient in casualty who has developed tetany. What is your management?

**150.** You confirm that an obese hypertensive patient has Cushing's syndrome. What are the possible causes?

**151.** What features would lead you to suspect that a comatose diabetic had lactic acidosis?

**152.** What are the indications for and dangers of oestrogen replacement therapy in post-menopausal women?

*Answers overleaf*

**149.** Reassurance

Sedation

Rebreathing into a bag which will terminate the attack and lead to a resolution of the tetany. This manoeuvre raises the $P_{CO_2}$ and corrects the respiratory alkalosis which has caused the tetany.

**150.** Adrenal hyperplasia—due to pituitary ACTH-producing adenomas or non-endocrine ACTH-producing tumour, e.g. bronchus, pancreas.

Adrenal tumours—either adenoma, or carcinoma.

Iatrogenic—corticosteroids, ACTH.

**151.** The patient was known to be taking a biguanide oral hypoglycaemic agent.

Evidence of acidosis clinically and biochemically.

Anion gap of greater than 12 mmol/l
(Calculate as $(Na^+ + K^+) - (Cl^- + HCO_3^-)$).

Absence of ketosis.

Confirmation by blood lactate level.

**152.** Possible indications are the alleviation of post menopausal problems of dyspareunia due to vaginal atrophy, hot flushes and the development of osteoporosis.

Absolute contraindications are previous breast or uterine carcinoma, or previous deep venous thrombosis, and relative contra-indications include family history of breast and uterine carcinoma, extensive endometriosis, cerebrovascular and coronary artery disease, diabetes mellitus, liver disease, hypertension, gallstones and pancreatitis. Alternative treatments such as oestrogen cream applied locally should be considered where appropriate. The dangers are mainly the 6–8 fold increase in endometrial carcinoma seen in oestrogen treated women. If oestrogen therapy is planned appropriate monitoring with pre-treatment endometrial biopsy, careful recording of medication and bleeding, regular breast and pelvic examinations and endometrial biopsy at regular intervals is necessary.

**153.** Outline the treatment of chronic adrenocortical insufficiency.

**154.** List the causes of adrenocortical insufficiency.

**155.** What features would lead you to suspect a diagnosis of carcinoid syndrome?

**156.** Summarize the management of diabetic ketoacidosis.

*Answers overleaf*

**153.** Replacement of glucocorticoid activity usually with cortisone acetate 37·5 mg daily.

Replacement of mineralocorticoid activity with fludrocortisone 0·1 mg daily.

Increase of dosage of cortisone during intercurrent illness and surgical operations.

**154.** Idiopathic (autoimmune)
Surgical removal
Previous corticosteroid therapy
Hypopituitarism
Infection, especially tuberculosis, fungal disease, syphilis
Haemorrhage into glands, usually a complication of (meningococcal) septicaemia
Others: bilateral tumour metastases, sarcoid, amyloid.

**155.** Cutaneous flushing of head and neck
Purple telangiectasia of these areas
Diarrhoea
Pulmonary stenosis and/or tricuspid incompetence.

One or more of the above, especially in association with hepatomegaly or other abdominal mass, merits consideration of the diagnosis.

**156.** Send off blood for gases, pH, plasma glucose, urea and electrolytes.

Commence i.v. infusion of normal saline (half normal if serum sodium is over 155 mmol/l or calculated osmolarity is over 330 mOsm/l) and aim to give 1·5–2 litres in the first 2 h; thereafter the rate of infusion depends on length of history, degree of dehydration and urine output. Infusion is changed to 5% dextrose when plasma glucose reaches 12 mmol/l. In the absence of renal failure or rising serum potassium, 20 mmol/hr potassium is added to the infusion fluid, although sometimes larger amounts are required.

Sodium bicarbonate is only necessary for severe acidosis (pH less than 7·0) or in renal failure.

Insulin is administered by infusion, initially 8 units per hour.

Aspirate stomach; given oxygen if patient is shocked; attach to cardiac monitor; monitor fluid balance.

Treat cause of decompensation, e.g. infection.

**157.** Thyrotoxic crisis or thyroid storm may develop postoperatively in patients poorly prepared for surgery or in thyrotoxic patients who develop some complicating medical illness. What is the management?

**158.** How would you treat Conn's syndrome (primary hyperaldosteronism?

**157.** General supportive measures include rehydration, provision of calories intravenously, nursing in a cooled humidified oxygen tent, and the use of a cooling blanket if hyperpyrexia is present.

Treat cardiac failure if present along usual lines.

Specific measures include large doses of antithyroid drugs e.g. propylthiouracil 100 mg every 2 h, iodine intravenously or orally, β-blockers and large doses of dexamethasone e.g. 2 mg 6-hourly.

**158.** If the cause is an adrenal adenoma:
Surgery is the treatment of choice; medical treatment with dietary salt restriction and spironolactone (for hypertension and hypokalaemia) is an alternative.

If the cause is bilateral adrenal hyperplasia:
Medical treatment with salt restriction and spironolactone is the treatment of choice.

# Gastroenterology and Hepatology

**159.** Is a normal liver palpable?

**160.** List some of the pathological causes of a palpable liver.

**161.** What is the significance of unconjugated hyperbilirubinaemia?

**162.** What does elevation of the serum transaminases mean?

**163.** What clotting factors are synthesized in the liver?

*Answers overleaf*

159. <u>Yes</u>; frequently in <u>childhood</u> or occasionally in <u>normal adults</u>, the liver edge is palpable below the right costal margin. A normal liver may have an extension of the right lobe palpable in the right flank—a Riedel's lobe; this is a normal variant. A normal sized liver may be displaced by an overexpanded chest as in <u>emphysema</u> or <u>acute asthma</u>, or by a <u>subphrenic lesion</u> such as an abscess.

160. Vascular congestion, e.g. congestive cardiac failure, hepatic vein obstruction
Biliary obstruction
Hepatitis
Cirrhosis (*Note:* many endstage cirrhotic livers are small and shrunken)
Tumours, cysts, abscess
Infiltration, e.g. leukaemia, lymphoma, amyloid, glycogen, fat, storage diseases, granulomas (e.g. sarcoid).

161. It indicates either excessive production of bilirubin because of haemolysis or a failure in hepatocyte uptake of unconjugated bilirubin, e.g. Gilbert's syndrome, hepatocyte necrosis.

162. It means that transaminase-containing cells are being damaged with consequent release of the enzymes into the blood. Aspartate aminotransferase (SGOT) is released from damaged hepatocytes, striated muscle cells, cardiac muscle cells, lung tissue and renal tissue. Alanine aminotransferase (SGPT) is released principally from damaged hepatocytes, therefore is a more useful marker of hepatocyte damage.

163. Fibrinogen, factors II, V, VII, IX and X. Production of factors II, VII, IX, X requires vitamin K. In hepatocellular failure the most likely factors to be affected are VII, II and X.

**164.** What viruses can cause acute hepatitis?

**165.** What are the symptoms and signs of portal hypertension?

**166.** Why do patients with liver failure get ascites?

**167.** List some of the cutaneous signs of chronic liver disease?

**168.** What can precipitate hepatic encephalopathy in a patient with cirrhosis?

*Answers overleaf*

**164.** Hepatitis A, B, non-A non-B viruses
Cytomegalovirus
Infectious mononucleosis (Epstein–Barr) virus
Yellow fever virus
Herpes simplex.

**165.** Symptoms — Gastrointestinal bleeding—especially haematemesis
from bleeding varices
Dyspepsia, epigastric pain and bloating
Abdominal and ankle swelling
Left upper quadrant pain (because of splenic
enlargement).

Signs — Ascites and oedema
Splenomegaly
Dilated abdominal veins
Haemorrhoids.

N.B. Portal hypertension may be present without symptoms or
signs.

**166.** Because of:
Portal hypertension
Lowered plasma oncotic pressure resulting from lowered plasma
albumin concentration
Failure to detoxify aldosterone in the damaged liver.

**167.** Jaundice
Spider naevi
Liver palms (palmar erythema)
White nails
Telangiectasia (paper money skin)
During skin examination, Dupuytren's contractures and parotid
swelling may be seen (especially in alcoholics) as well as
gynaecomastia.

**168.** High protein meal
GI bleed
Hypokalaemia
Extreme diuresis
Injudicious paracentesis abdominis
Opiates, barbiturates or other sedative drugs, alcohol
Infection.

**169.** Outline your treatment of hepatic ascites.

**170.** Outline your management of bleeding oesophageal varices.

**171.** In which liver diseases are steroids indicated?

**172.** What is cirrhosis?

*Answers overleaf*

**169.** Bed rest

Dietary salt restriction (to c.22 mmol/day)

Fluid restriction (to 1 litre/day)

If these measures fail, cautiously start a potassium-sparing diuretic (e.g. spironolactone, amiloride) with daily monitoring of plasma urea and electrolytes, urine output, abdominal girth and body weight. Ideal weight loss—1 kg/day. If still no diuresis, cautiously start a loop diuretic (e.g. frusemide)—this can cause hypokalaemia or uraemia and precipitate encephalopathy.

Paracentesis is never used as a treatment of hepatic ascites.

**170.** I.V. line; check haemoglobin, urea, electrolytes, prothrombin time and platelet count; cross match blood.

Resuscitate patient with fresh blood and, if indicated, fresh frozen plasma.

Confirm diagnosis with endoscopy.

If bleeding recurs or continues, consider vasopressin infusion, oesophageal tamponade.

If bleeding continues in spite of above measures, consider sclerotherapy. In the last resort, a surgical procedure such as oesophageal transection or emergency portacaval shunt should be considered.

**171.** Usually:

Chronic active hepatitis (Hepatitis B antigen negative)

Sometimes:

Chronic active hepatitis (Hepatitis B antigen positive)

Prolonged cholestasis in acute viral hepatitis

Controversially:

Acute alcoholic hepatitis

Acute fulminant hepatic failure.

**172.** Cirrhosis is defined pathologically and is a diffuse abnormality of liver characterized by fibrosis and a conversion of normal architecture into structurally abnormal nodules. Both nodules and fibrosis must be present to make the diagnosis.

**173.** What types of liver disease are particularly associated with the development of hepatic cell carcinoma?

**174.** List some of the causes of cirrhosis?

**175.** List some of the causes of bleeding per rectum.

**176.** Outline the treatment of irritable bowel syndrome.

*Answers overleaf*

**173.** Hepatitis B associated liver disease
Haemochromatosis

**174.** Cryptogenic
Infections—viral hepatitis
Autoimmune—chronic active hepatitis
        primary biliary cirrhosis
Drugs and toxins—alcohol
        methyldopa
Biliary obstruction
Vascular—chronic right ventricular failure
      constrictive pericarditis
      hepatic vein occlusion
Metabolic—Wilson's disease
      haemochromatosis
      $\alpha_1$-antitrypsin deficiency.

**175.** Haemorrhoids
Carcinoma of large bowel
Diverticulosis
Colonic polyps
Inflammatory bowel disease (ulcerative colitis, Crohn's disease)
Dysentery—shigella
      amoebic
Rectal ulcer
Proctitis—idiopathic
     radiation
     infection, e.g. gonorrhoea
Ischaemic colitis.

N.B. Upper G.I. tract bleeding may lead to passage of fresh blood
P.R. if the haemorrhage is torrential.

**176.** Explanation and reassurance
High fibre diet
Additional medication as indicated: for constipation, e.g. sterculia or
frangula, lactulose; for severe pain—antispasmodics, e.g.
mebeverine, clidinium; for anxiety e.g. diazepam. For those with
painless diarrhoea only, codeine phosphate or equivalent may be
indicated.

177. What types of colonic inflammatory disease do you know?

178. What is proctalgia fugax?

179. If a patient presents with a perianal abscess, should you consider underlying disease?

180. Do any conditions predispose to carcinoma of the colon?

181. Which part of the large intestine is the commonest site for carcinoma?

182. What is the prognosis of colonic cancer?

*Answers overleaf*

**177.** Idiopathic—ulcerative colitis
　　Crohn's disease
　Infection, e.g. shigellosis
　　　salmonellosis
　　　amoebiasis
　　　*Clostridium difficile* associated colitis
　　　Campylobacter colitis
　Ischaemic colitis

**178.** Severe attacks of rectal pain in the absence of organic disease. Most sufferers are young or middle-aged males and the attacks are frequently nocturnal, lasting up to 15 min.

**179.** Yes—Crohn's disease, tuberculosis, immune deficiency and neutropenia.

**180.** Adenoma (particularly villous adenoma)
　Ulcerative colitis (and ?Crohn's colitis)
　Familial polyposis coli
　Gardner's syndrome (variant of polyposis coli with osteomas and soft-tissue tumours).

**181.** Rectum—almost one-third of cases. Other sites in order of frequency: sigmoid colon, descending colon, caecum, ascending colon, transverse colon, splenic and hepatic flexure.

**182.** Of all patients operated upon, 5-year survival is 45%. However, survival is related to extent of spread which is expressed by Dukes staging:
Stage A (tumour confined to bowel wall, no metastases)—80% 5-year survival.
Stage B (tumour penetrating wall no metastases)—60% 5-year survival.
Stage C (regional lymph node metastases)—30% 5-year survival.
Stage D (distant metastases)—5% 5-year survival.

**183.** What disorders might cause chronic constipation?

**184.** What are the main histological types of oesophageal carcinoma?

**185.** What are the common symptoms of gastric carcinoma?

*Answers overleaf*

**183.** Simple rectal constipation (habitual failure to answer the urge to defaecate)
Diverticulosis
Irritable bowel syndrome
Colonic carcinoma
Bowel obstruction
Megacolon—congenital (Hirschsprung's disease)
        acquired
Painful perianal conditions
Depression
Anorexia nervosa
Pelvic trauma, pregnancy, etc.
Weakness of perineal musculature—ageing, neurological disease
Metabolic—hypothyroidism
            hypercalcaemia
            porphyria
Toxins—lead
Drugs—opiates.

**184.** Squamous carcinoma—95%
Adenocarcinoma

N.B. Many lower oesophageal carcinomas are in fact fundal gastric carcinomas.

**185.** Epigastric pain; dyspepsia
Weight loss
Anorexia
Vomiting
Early satiety
Dysphagia (in fundal lesions)
Gastrointestinal bleeding—acute
                            chronic
Weakness.

**186.** What are the possible sequelae of gallstones?

**187.** How would you dissolve gallstones medically?

**188.** What symptoms would lead you to suspect the presence of gallstone disease?

**189.** What is a Crosby capsule?

**190.** What are the main histological features of the jejunal mucosa in untreated coeliac disease?

*Answers overleaf*

**186.** None—the patient is asymptomatic
Cystic duct obstruction leading to acute cholecystitis
Biliary obstruction leading to obstructive jaundice and possibly cholangitis and cirrhosis
Chronic cholecystitis
Acute pancreatitis—results from stones in the common bile duct
Carcinoma of the gallbladder—90% of cases have gall stones
Gall stone ileus—results from a stone passing through a cholecysto-intestinal fistula which is caused by acute cholecystitis with perforation of the gallbladder into adherent small bowel.

**187.** Cholesterol-containing stones without evidence of calcification may be dissolved by ursodeoxycholic or chenodeoxycholic acid taken by mouth. The stones have to be less than 15 mm in diameter and the gallbladder has to function.

**188.** Right upper quadrant pain with or without fever
Obstructive jaundice
Flatulence, dyspepsia, epigastric pain, vomiting
Cholangitic symptoms, i.e. fever, right upper quadrant pain and jaundice.

**189.** A small device approximately 1 cm in length which, attached to a length of radiopaque tubing, is passed into the jejunum to obtain a jejunal biopsy. The capsule contains a spring loaded blade which is triggered by suction when the jejunal mucosa overlies an orifice across which the blade passes.

**190.** Flattening and broadening of the villi to give a flat mucosa (so-called subtotal villous atrophy).
Increased crypt depth
Cuboidal epithelial cells
Mononuclear cell infiltration of the lamina propria and epithelium.

**191.** List the important causes of chronic diarrhoea?

**192.** What is double-contrast radiology of the GI tract?

**193.** What are the advantages of endoscopy of the GI tract over radiology?

**194.** What is the Mallory–Weiss syndrome?

*Answers overleaf*

**191.** 

| Inflammatory | Infection |
|---|---|
| Crohn's disease | Tuberculosis (rare) |
| Ulcerative colitis | Amoebiasis |
| Drugs | Giardiasis |
| Especially antibiotics, | Endocrine |
| laxatives | Hyperthyroidism |
| Tumour | Vipoma (rare) |
| Carcinoma | Zollinger–Ellison Syndrome |
| Villous adenoma | (rare) |
| Malabsorption | Neurological |
| Small intestinal | Postvagotomy |
| Pancreatic | Diabetes |
| Intestinal resection | Irritable Bowel Syndrome |

**192.** More information and greater detail is available when gas is introduced into the stomach or large bowel in addition to barium. Effervescent tablets are used in a double-contrast barium meal. These distend the stomach and enable a fine coating of barium to show up small lesions such as erosions or small polyps. Similarly a barium enema is improved with the addition of gas, distending the large bowel and enabling small ulcers, polyps, neoplasms and other mucosal lesions to be identified.

**193.** Visualization of small mucosal lesions which may be missed using double-contrast radiology.
Visualization of active bleeding, or evidence of recent bleeding.
The facility to take cytological and histological specimens.
Its use in therapeutic procedures such as oesophageal dilatation, injection of oesophageal varices or polypectomy.

**194.** Laceration of the mucosa in the region of the gastro-oesophageal junction. There is characteristically a history of retching or vomiting followed by haematemesis. With the advent of endoscopy the incidence of this condition, about 10% of all upper gastro-intestinal bleeds, was found to be greater than previously thought.

**195.** What are the symptoms of reflux oesophagitis?

**196.** What treatment is available for achalasia?

**197.** Why is the death rate from gastric cancer declining?

**198.** How may the gastrointestinal tract be involved in progressive systemic sclerosis?

*Answers overleaf*

**195.**   The main symptom of reflux oesophagitis, which may be present with or without an associated hiatal hernia, is oesophageal mucosal pain. This is typically a retrosternal burning pain but may be felt at, and radiate to, other sites. It is provoked by reflux which most often occurs after the ingestion of food, while wearing tight clothing, or on bending down. The pain is often troublesome at night when the supine position predisposes to reflux. Acid regurgitation, felt as a bitter taste in the mouth, may occur. Some patients remain asymptomatic but may present later with an oesophageal stricture.

**196.**   Drugs—nitrates, calcium antagonists—may be helpful symptomatically but have no place in the definitive management.

Surgery—oesophagomyotomy (Heller's operation)—probably the treatment of choice. The lower oesophageal sphincter is incised.

Pneumatic dilatation—lower oesophageal sphincter fibres are torn by forceful dilatation with a pneumatic bag.

**197.**   Because the incidence of the condition itself is falling (for reasons unknown). No improvements in surgical results have been obtained; 5-year survival is still less than 10%. An exception to this is the small number of patients with early gastric cancer, diagnosed endoscopically, who have a good prognosis.

**198.**   Mouth—puckering and narrowing leading to 'microstoma' and difficulty in mastication.
Oesophagus—weakening of gastro-oesophageal sphincter leading to reflux oesophagitis and stricture; loss of oesophageal motility.
Stomach—delay in gastric emptying and atony (rare).
Small intestine—atonic segments leading to bacterial overgrowth and malabsorption.
Large intestine—large square shaped diverticula.
Liver—there is an association with primary biliary cirrhosis.

**199.** What is the Zollinger–Ellison syndrome?

**200.** What are the complications of duodenal ulcer?

**201.** Give the significance and the causes of dysphagia.

*Answers overleaf*

**199.** The production of excessive amounts of gastrin by an islet cell tumour of the pancreas or G-cell tumour of the duodenum. 60% of gastrinomas are malignant. The diagnosis should be suspected when:

There is failure of a duodenal ulcer to heal.

A recurrent ulcer occurs after surgery.

Multiple ulcers are found in a young person.

The diagnosis is confirmed by the finding of a greatly elevated serum gastrin.

**200.** Haemorrhage—may occur in up to 20% of patients with duodenal ulcer over a 25-year period.

Perforation—may occur in approximately 6% of patients with duodenal ulcer.

Pyloric stenosis.

**201.** Dysphagia, or difficulty in swallowing, is an important symptom usually indicating organic disease or dysfunction. It should not be confused with globus hystericus, the sensation of a lump in the throat independent of swallowing, and usually emotional in origin. For ease of classification the causes can be divided into those

Within the lumen:

carcinoma

stricture

oesophageal ring.

Within the wall:

diffuse oesophageal spasm

achalasia

scleroderma—dysphagia usually caused by peptic stricture secondary to reflux oesophagitis.

Outside the wall:

aortic or cardiac aneurysm

vascular anomalies

mediastinal tumours

large left atrium

para-oesophageal diaphragmatic hernia.

Oropharyngeal disorders, which are most commonly due to neuromuscular disorders, may also cause dysphagia by inhibition of the initiation of swallowing.

**202.** How is possible malabsorption of fat assessed?

**203.** What is the xylose absorption test?

**204.** What tests may be helpful in the diagnosis of lactose intolerance?

**205.** What is a gluten-free diet, what are the sources of gluten and in what condition is it the main treatment?

*Answers overleaf*

**202.** The best method is by direct measurement of faecal fat in a three-day stool collection while on a standard 70–100 g fat intake diet. Excretion greater than 20 mmol/day is considered abnormal. Indirect methods are unreliable.

**203.** A test used to assess carbohydrate absorption from the jejunum. 25 g of xylose (a monosaccharide) is administered orally and urine collected for 5 hours. This should contain a minimum of 4·5 g xylose. Measurement of blood xylose, after 1 or 2 hours, obviates the difficulties of renal excretion and urine collection, but does not avoid the artificially low values due to delayed gastric emptying.

**204.** Lactose tolerance test—where the rise in plasma glucose is monitored after ingestion of a standard amount of lactose.

Lactose hydrogen breath test—excretion of breath $H_2$ increases when unabsorbed lactose comes into contact with the bacteria of the colon.

Lactose barium meal—ingestion of lactose with barium causes oedema and dilatation of the proximal small bowel if lactose intolerance is present.

Jejunal brush border lactase—activity is measured in a jejunal biopsy specimen—it does not always correlate with clinical lactose intolerance.

N.B. Oral lactose tests may be associated with the production of abdominal pain and diarrhoea if lactose intolerance is present.

**205.** A gluten-free diet excludes a group of protein substances which can be separated from wheat, rye, barley or oat flour. Gluten may be contained in many unlikely proprietary foods, e.g. sweets, ice-cream, and in certain drugs, e.g. Dimotane. It is used in the treatment of coeliac disease.

**206.** What is the commonest cause of a patient with coeliac disease failing to respond to a gluten-free diet?

**207.** What are the long-term complications of partial gastrectomy?

**208.** What are the causes of upper gastrointestinal haemorrhage?

**209.** What is your first course of action in the management of a patient who has been admitted in shock due to gastrointestinal haemorrhage?

*Answers overleaf*

**206.** Failure to adhere strictly, often inadvertently, to a gluten-free diet.

Other causes include lactase deficiency, intestinal ulceration and lymphoma.

N.B. About 10% of adult coeliacs fail to respond to a strict gluten free diet.

**207.** Small stomach remnant leading to early satiety and weight loss.
Rapid bowel transit.
Iron deficiency.
$B_{12}$ deficiency.
Osteomalacia.
Unmasking of coeliac disease or lactase deficiency.
Bacterial overgrowth of the small intestine.

**208.** Duodenal ulcer
Gastritis
Gastric or duodenal erosions
Gastric ulcer
Oesophagitis
Mallory–Weiss tear
Gastric carcinoma
Oesophageal varices
Oesophageal carcinoma
Rare causes such as leiomyoma, Osler–Weber–Rendu syndrome, bleeding disorders, acute aneurysm, angiodysplasia, pseudoxanthoma elasticum.

**209.** Put up an intravenous infusion and commence a plasma volume expander.
Blood for cross-matching and haemoglobin should be taken at the same time.

**210.** In establishing a diagnosis of ulcerative colitis, is it sufficient to obtain a rectal biopsy with histology reported as showing typical features of the conditions? What are the typical features?

**211.** List the extra-intestinal complications of ulcerative colitis.

**212.** What areas of the gastrointestinal tract may be affected by Crohn's disease?

**213.** What drugs are used in the treatment of ulcerative colitis?

*Answers overleaf*

**210.** The typical histological features are infiltration of polymorphs and plasma cells into the lamina propria with vascular dilatation and oedema, crypt abscess formation, goblet cell depletion, glandular destruction and ulceration of the surface epithelium.

Although the history will usually suggest the diagnosis of ulcerative colitis, bacterial infections and Crohn's disease may show similar histological features, although in Crohn's disease, transmural submucosal inflammation and non-caseating granulomas are more usually found. Therefore further investigation such as radiology, stool microscopy and culture are essential.

**211.** Apththous ulceration
Skin—erythema nodosum, pyoderma gangrenosum
Joints—acute arthritis (linked to disease activity); sacro-iliitis and ankylosing spondylitis (unrelated to disease activity)
Eyes—conjunctivitis, episcleritis, uveitis
Liver/biliary—pericholangitis, sclerosing chlolangitis, bile duct carcinoma, chronic active hepatitis, cirrhosis.

**212.** Crohn's disease may affect any part of the gastrointestinal tract from mouth to anus. It more commonly occurs in the terminal ileum, caecum, rectum and perineal region, colon, proximal ileum and jejunum but less frequently in duodenum, stomach and oesophagus.

**213.** Corticosteroids—may be given orally, topically (by enema) or in severe cases, intravenously. They suppress inflammation during acute exacerbations, but are of no value in preventing relapse.

Sulphasalazine—is used mainly to maintain remission but it may be used to suppress mild inflammatory activity. It is usually given orally but can be given by enema.

Azathioprine—is occasionally used in those not responding to conventional treatment and to reduce the dose of systemic steroids.

**214.** List the causes of acute pancreatitis.

**215.** Summarize the treatment of chronic pancreatitis.

**216.** What is the significance of a raised serum amylase?
Should an attack of acute pancreatitis be treated by physicians or surgeons?

**217.** What types of gallstones do you know?

*Answers overleaf*

**214.** Alcohol
Gallstones
Metabolic disorders—hyperparathyroidism
    hyperlipidaemia
Abdominal trauma
Postoperative
Post ERCP
Mumps
Drugs including thiazides, frusemide, azathioprine, sulphasalazine,
    steroids, tetracycline
Hereditary.

**215.** Withdraw alcohol, remove gallstones.
Treat painful attacks with admission to hospital, nasogastric suction,
    analgesics, depending on severity of attack.
Treat diabetes with diet, oral hypoglycaemic agents or insulin as
    necessary. Acute diabetes during a severe attack may be self
    limiting and require no treatment.
Treat steatorrhoea and nutritional problems with low fat diet,
    pancreatic enzyme supplements taken with meals 30 min after $H_2$
    receptor antagonist, and medium-chain triglyceride supplements.
Surgery may be indicated for severe pain or pseudocyst.

**216.** A raised serum amylase above 1000 Somogyi units is strong
    evidence in favour of pancreatitis but lower levels, although
    elevated above normal, may be associated with other intra-
    abdominal pathology, e.g. intestinal perforation, obstruction or
    infarction, cholecystitis, hepatitis, ruptured ectopic pregnancy,
    uraemia.

The treatment of uncomplicated acute pancreatitis is medical but in
    the case of presentation as an acute abdomen a laparotomy may
    be considered necessary for diagnostic purposes.

**217.** Solitary cholesterol stone—containing more than 95%
    cholesterol.
Mixed cholesterol stones containing over 70% cholesterol but also
    calcium salts, bile acids and pigments, fatty acids and
    phospholipids.
Pigment stones, about 20% of gallstones, containing no cholesterol
    are made up of bilirubin. In UK there is often an association with
    chronic haemolytic anaemia or hepatic cirrhosis.

**218.** What symptoms are caused by peptic ulceration?

**219.** List the side effects of antacids.

**220.** What drugs have been shown to heal duodenal ulcer?

**221.** Do all peptic ulcers heal with cimetidine?

*Answers overleaf*

**218.** Abdominal pain—usually epigastric or sometimes right hypo-chondrial. Periodicity with spontaneous remission for days or weeks is characteristic. Relationship to food is variable but nocturnal pain is typical of duodenal ulcer.

Vomiting—may be prominent in those with pyloric channel ulceration.

Weight loss—especially with gastric ulcers. Weight gain may occur in those obtaining relief by eating.

Heartburn, acid regurgitation, excessive salivation, and eructation may also be described.

**219.** Diarrhoea (magnesium salts)
Constipation (aluminium salts)
Acid rebound (calcium salts)
Milk alkali syndrome—caused by ingestion of large quantities of calcium, usually in the form of milk, and antacids, especially sodium bicarbonate, which cause alkalosis.

Hypophosphataemia—caused by aluminium binding phosphate in the intestine.

Oedema and sodium retention—in patients with cardiac failure or hepatic ascites who are given antacids containing excessive sodium.

**220.** Drugs inhibiting acid output:
$H_2$ receptor antagonists, e.g. cimetidine
Pirenzepine
Trimipramine
Prostaglandin $E_2$.

Drugs neutralizing acid output:
Aluminium—magnesium liquid antacids in large doses.

Drugs increasing mucosal resistance:
Carbenoxolone (as Duogastrone)
Tripotasso-dicitrato bismuthate (De Nol)
Sucralfate.

**221.** No; about 80% of chronic duodenal ulcers heal on cimetidine in standard dose (1 g/day) over 6 weeks compared to 25–40% on placebo treatment. Figures for gastric ulcer are less clear but probably about 50–60% of gastric ulcers will heal with cimetidine over 6 weeks compared to 40–50% with placebo therapy.

# Haematology

**222.** Define anaemia.

**223.** What are the sites of $B_{12}$ and folate absorption?

**224.** What are the causes of iron deficiency anaemia?

**225.** What tests suggest and confirm that haemolysis is taking place?

**226.** What is the anaemia of chronic disease?

**227.** List the causes of aplastic anaemia.

*Answers overleaf*

**222.** Anaemia is a reduction in haemoglobin concentration with or without a decrease in red cell numbers.

**223.** $B_{12}$—specific as receptors for $B_{12}$-intrinsic factor complex in the ileum.
Folate—largely absorbed in the proximal jejunum--the mechanism of absorption is controversial.

**224.** Poor diet
Pregnancy and lactation
Blood loss—acute
           chronic
Malabsorption.

**225.** Anaemia—normochromic and normocytic; occasionally macrocytic
Reticulocytosis
Unconjugated hyperbilirubinaemia
Urobilinogenuria
Erythroid hyperplasia in the bone marrow
Reduced or absent serum haptoglobin
Methaemalbuminaemia (intravascular haemolysis)
Haemoglobinuria (intravascular haemolysis)
Haemosiderinuria (intravascular haemolysis)
Reduced red cell survival.

**226.** The normochromic, normocytic anaemia seen in such disorders as chronic sepsis, chronic inflammatory disease, e.g. rheumatoid arthritis, malignant disease and uraemia.

**227.** Primary (idiopathic)
Secondary
    Drugs, e.g. chloramphenicol, phenylbutazone, cytotoxics, antimetabolites.
    Toxins, e.g. benzol and derivatives
    Radiation
    Marrow replacement by fibrosis, tumour or other abnormal cells.

**228.** What are the common indications for a bone marrow examination?

**229.** What is a leukaemic leukaemia?

**230.** What types of leukaemia are associated with chromosomal abnormalities?

**231.** Is any form of leukaemia curable?

**232.** What are the clinical features of chronic myeloid leukaemia?

*Answers overleaf*

**228.** Unexplained anaemia
Suspected aplastic anaemia
Granulocytopenia
Thrombocytopenia
Suspected marrow replacement with tumour, leukaemic cells, myeloma cells, fibrosis.
Disseminated infection, e.g. T.B. in which bone marrow is cultured.

**229.** An acute leukaemia with no blast cells in the peripheral blood. It is diagnosed on bone marrow examination.

**230.** Chronic myeloid leukaemia—especially the Philadelphia chromosome—seen in 90% of cases.

Acute myeloblastic leukaemia—especially in the acute promyelocytic variety in which translocations may be seen.

**231.** There is increasing evidence that acute lymphoblastic leukaemia in children may be curable in some cases.

**232.** Majority of patients are 30–50 years old.
Left upper quadrant pain (because of splenomegaly and/or splenic infarction)
Symptoms of anaemia
Weight loss
Fever
Massive splenomegaly
Bleeding manifestations.

**233.** Give a differential diagnosis of neutropenia (granulocytopenia).

**234.** What causes death in acute leukaemia?

**235.** What is purpura?

**236.** What are the major types of bleeding disorder?

**237.** What investigations would you do to exclude a bleeding disorder?

*Answers overleaf*

**233.** Drug-induced neutropenia, e.g. chloramphenicol, phenothiazines, carbamazepine, carbimazole, propylthiouracil, cytotoxics, antimetabolites.

Blood diseases, e.g. chronic idiopathic neutropenia, cyclical neutropenia, leukaemia, pancytopenia.

Nutritional deficiencies, e.g. $B_{12}$, folate (especially in alcoholics).

Secondary to infections, e.g. typhoid, infectious mononucleosis, overwhelming sepsis.

Splenic enlargement—hypersplenism.

Malignant infiltration of bone marrow.

Felty's syndrome.

**234.** Progressive anaemia, infection and bleeding (especially intracerebral) because infiltration of marrow leads to aplastic anaemia, neutropenia and thrombocytopenia; These may be caused or aggravated by cytotoxic therapy.

Leukaemic meningitis, especially in patients whose blood and marrow remit but who did not receive adequate prophylactic C.N.S. irradiation or cytotoxic therapy.

**235.** Purpura is bleeding into the skin or mucous membranes. It is a sign not a disease. It does not blanche with pressure and exhibits the colour changes of a bruise as it fades. Pin point purpuric spots are petechiae; larger areas of purpura are ecchymoses (or bruises).

**236.** Platelet deficiency
Increased capillary fragility
Defects in mechanisms of clotting.

**237.** Hess' test
Bleeding time
Whole blood clotting time
Platelet count
Prothrombin time
Thrombin time
Activated partial thromboplastin time.

**238.** What is hypersplenism?

**239.** List some of the causes of splenomegaly.

**240.** In what blood disorders may splenectomy commonly be indicated?

*Answers overleaf*

**238.** It is a syndrome of splenomegaly (from any cause) associated with pancytopenia and a hyperplastic marrow. The blood picture returns to normal after splenectomy.

**239.** Portal hypertension
Blood diseases
    Chronic iron deficiency
    Pernicious anaemia
    Haemolytic anaemias
    Thalassaemias
    Leukaemias
    Lymphomas
    Myelofibrosis
    Polycythaemia rubra vera
Infections, e.g.
    Septicaemia
    Brucellosis
    Malaria
    T.B.
    Infectious mononucleosis
    Infective hepatitis
    Kala-azar
    Subacute infective endocarditis
Others
    Felty's syndrome
    Systemic lupus erythematosus
    Sarcoidosis
    Cysts and tumours
    Storage diseases, e.g. Gaucher's disease.

**240.** Hereditary spherocytosis and elliptocytosis
Idiopathic thrombocytopenic purpura
Autoimmune haemolytic anaemia
Hypersplenism.

**241.** What is the differential diagnosis of generalised lymphadenopathy?

**242.** Which generally has the better prognosis, Hodgkins or non-Hodgkins lymphoma?

**243.** What is the commonest cause of anaemia in Great Britain?

**244.** What types of polycythaemia are there?

**245.** How would you treat polycythaemia rubra vera?

*Answers overleaf*

**241.** Neoplasia, e.g.
   leukaemias
   lymphomas
Infections, e.g.
   infectious mononucleosis
   brucellosis
   toxoplasmosis
   cytomegalovirus
   rubella
   Whipple's disease
   syphilis
Inflammatory disorders, e.g.
   serum sickness
   sarcoidosis
   rheumatoid arthritis
   systemic lupus erythematosus
Storage diseases, e.g.
   Gaucher's disease
Drugs, e.g.
   phenytoin
Extensive exfoliative skin rashes (dermatopathic lymphadenitis).

**242.** Hodgkin's disease; even in advanced disease (Stages III and IV) 80% of patients completely remit and 65% of these remain disease free at 10 years.

**243.** Iron-deficiency anaemia.

**244.** Primary polycythaemia = polycythaemia rubra vera
Secondary polycythaemia
Relative polycythaemia—the result of a decrease in plasma volume because of dehydration and haemoconcentration.

**245.** Venesection is now the basis of treatment in most cases. It is probably as good as marrow suppression with busulphan, chlorambucil or melphalan. Marrow suppression with radioactive $^{32}$P is also effective but is associated with an increased risk of developing acute leukaemia. Gout may be precipitated by treatment, so allopurinol 300 mg/day should be given during treatment.

**246.** Why is allopurinol frequently prescribed for patients undergoing cytotoxic therapy for lymphoma and neoplastic diseases of the blood?

**247.** What is the average Western daily dietary intake of iron and in what foods is it found?

**248.** What complication of blood transfusion do you know?

**249.** Under what physiological conditions is there a risk of developing iron-deficiency anaemia?

**250.** What is transferrin?

**251.** What is haemoglobin F and what percentage of total adult haemoglobin does it constitute?

*Answers overleaf*

**246.** Destruction of large numbers of neoplastic cells by the cytotoxic drugs leads to substantial release of purines and pyrimidines which are then converted to uric acid. Therefore acute gout can be precipitated. Allopurinol is given at the start of chemotherapy to prevent formation of uric acid and to prevent gout.

**247.** 10–20 mg daily in such foods as meat, particularly liver. A small amount is contained in cereals and bread, and vegetables.

**248.** Immune mediated reactions
    Intravascular haemolysis—usually due to ABO incompatability
    Extravascular haemolysis—usually due to Rhesus incompatability
    Febrile reactions due to minor immunity to white cell, platelet or plasma antigens.

Non-immune reactions
    Circulatory overload
    Transmission of infection, e.g. malaria, hepatitis B, syphilis
    Air and fat embolism
    Thrombophlebitis
    Hyperkalaemia, citrate toxicity and dilutional coagulopathy as a result of massive transfusion of stored blood.
    Haemosiderosis as a result of multiple transfusions.

**249.** Menstrual losses in excess of 80 ml monthly
Pregnancy
Teenage pubertal growth spurt.

**250.** A serum glycoprotein of molecular weight about 80 000 which specifically binds iron and is responsible for its delivery to the tissues.

**251.** Haemoglobin F is the major haemoglobin during fetal life and is made up of $2\alpha$ and $2\gamma$ chains. It constitutes between 50 and 90% of the total haemoglobin at birth and decreases progressively to less than 1% by the age of one year (with an associated reciprocal rise in HbA).

**252.** What conditions lead to a microcytic blood film?

**253.** What are the main approaches to treatment in thalassaemia?

**254.** What are the clinical features of thalassaemia major?

**255.** Outline the management of sickle-cell anaemia.

**256.** What does the level of haptoglobin in the blood indicate?

*Answers overleaf*

**252.** Microcytosis may be present in iron deficiency, thalassaemia, anaemia of chronic disease, lead poisoning, thyrotoxicosis, sideroblastic anaemia and hereditary spherocytosis.

**253.** Red cell transfusion
Iron chelation to reduce haemosiderosis (desferrioxamine)
Treat infections promptly
Give folic acid when indicated
Delay splenectomy for gross splenomegaly or severe hypersplenism until late childhood because of increased risk of pneumococcal septicaemia.

**254.** Anaemia
Marked skeletal deformities due to bone-marrow expansion with frontal bossing, distortion of ribs and vertebrae and pathological fracture of long bones
Progressive hepatosplenomegaly and hypersplenism
Gallstones
Chronic leg ulcers
Retarded growth and sexual development
Intercurrent infections
Haemosiderosis after repeated transfusion leading to cardiac, pancreatic or hepatic insufficiency.

**255.** Prompt recognition and treatment of infections } both of which are contributory
Correction of folate deficiency } factors in 'aplastic crises'
Red cell transfusion or exchange transfusion (replacing about 50% of the patient's blood) for severe anaemia, or as a means of preventing painful vaso-occlusive crises.
Manage painful crises by vigorous hydration, analgesics, oxygen, correction of acidosis and treatment of infection. Hypertonic oxygen and antiplatelet agents may be useful.

**256.** Haptoglobin forms complexes with free haemoglobin released by haemolysis and is removed by the reticuloendothelial system. Hence reduction in haptoglobin levels is strong evidence for haemolysis. Haptoglobin is an acute phase reactant and is increased in inflammatory or infective conditions.

**257.** What are the clinical features of anaemia irrespective of underlying abnormality?

**258.** What is koilonychia?

**259.** What are the three main factors concerned with the arrest of haemorrhage?

**260.** What is the more descriptive name for the eponymous Osler–Weber–Rendu syndrome and what are the main clinical features?

**261.** What haematological abnormalities are characteristic of von Willebrand's disease?

**262.** What is the defect in classic haemophilia (haemophilia A)?

**263.** What blood products are used in the management of haemophilia A?

*Answers overleaf*

**257.** Fatigue, lassitude and weakness, dyspnoea on exertion, dizziness, faintness, headache, insomnia, dyspepsia, an unmasking or exacerbation of angina pectoris, pallor of skin and mucous membranes, palpitations, tachycardia, systolic murmur and sometimes frank cardiac failure with pulmonary and ankle oedema.

**258.** Koilonychia refers to changes occurring in the nails in chronic iron deficiency, manifest first by brittleness and dryness and later flattening and thinning of the nails. Finally the nails become concave, so-called spoon-shaped nails.

**259.** The vascular factor, with contraction of damaged small vessels.
The platelet factor, with the aggregation of platelets and plugging of the bleeding points in the vessels.
The coagulation factor, with initiation of the 'clotting cascade' leading to the formation of fibrin.

**260.** Hereditary haemorrhagic telangiectasia
Autosomal dominant inheritance; multiple telangiectasia especially of face and mucous membranes; epistaxis, haematemesis, haemoptysis (from pulmonary A–V malformations) and haematuria.

**261.** Capillary abnormality with prolonged bleeding time.
Reduced level of factor VIII in some cases.
Abnormal platelet function.

**262.** Reduced levels of factor VIII coagulant which is inherited as a sex-linked recessive characteristic.

**263.** Cryoprecipitate, manufactured by blood banks and stored frozen.
Factor VIII concentrates, stored in lyophilised form and brought into solution by adding water.
Fresh frozen plasma is suitable, but is rarely used.

**264.** How would you investigate a patient who presents with a megaloblastic anaemia?

**265.** List the differential diagnosis of macrocytosis on a peripheral blood film other than megaloblastic anaemia.

**266.** What are the causes of secondary polycythaemia?

**267.** Pulmonary infiltrates seen on chest X-ray, parasitic infection with worms, polyarteritis nodosa and Hodgkin's disease may have what abnormality in common in the peripheral blood film?

**268.** What is the significance of a positive direct Coombs' test in haemolytic anaemia?

**269.** What is the significance of an increased reticulocyte count in the peripheral blood film?

*Answers overleaf*

**264.** Measure serum $B_{12}$ and red cell folate levels (but the latter may be low in pure $B_{12}$ deficiency).

$B_{12}$ deficiency:
Note points in history particularly in relation to diet, drugs, previous surgery, visits to tropics and family history.
Schilling test—Part I to determine whether $B_{12}$ malabsorption is present and part II to determine if it is improved by intrinsic factor.
Malabsorption of $B_{12}$ uncorrected by intrinsic factor requires further investigation with particular consideration of bacterial overgrowth or terminal ileum disease.

Folate deficiency:
History in relation to diet is particularly important, as is drug history.
Proximal small intestinal diseases, especially coeliac disease, must be considered and investigated accordingly.

**265.** Alcohol excess, liver disease, myxoedema, leucoerythroblastic anaemia, cytotoxic drug therapy, pregnancy, haemolysis.

**266.** Chronic respiratory disease, heart lesions producing right-to-left shunts, high affinity haemoglobins, carboxyhaemoglobinaemia, renal cysts and hydronephrosis, renal carcinoma, hepatoma, cerebellar haemangioblastoma, massive uterine fibroids, androgen-secreting tumours, phaeochromocytoma, high altitude.

**267.** All these conditions may have a raised eosinophil count, which may also be caused by drug reactions.

**268.** It indicates an autoimmune basis. Further tests are indicated to determine if the haemolysis is primary or secondary to drugs or some underlying disorder.

**269.** Reticulocytosis indicates release of increased numbers of young red cells from the bone marrow and is a feature of increased erythropoiesis. A significant elevation of the reticulocyte count occurs in haemolysis, haemorrhage, in the response to haematinics in deficiency anaemias, and in patients with leucoerythroblastic anaemia.

**270.** What investigations would you perform to confirm suspected disseminated intravascular coagulation (DIC)?

**271.** What are the clinical features of acute leukaemia?

**272.** What are the indications for treatment in an elderly patient with chronic lymphatic leukaemia (CLL)?

**273.** How would a reaction due to a mismatched blood transfusion present?

*Answers overleaf*

270. Fibrinogen level which is low.
Measurement of fibrin and fibrinogen degradation products (FDP) which are increased.
The ethanol gelatin and protamine sulphate precipitation tests which are positive when there are circulating fibrin molecules even before clot formation.
Thrombin clotting time which is increased because of interference by FDP.
The platelet count which is reduced.

271. They are the consequences of bone marrow failure with anaemia (pallor, palpitations, weakness and dyspnoea) neutropenia (infection, especially of mouth and chest, and septicaemia) and thrombocytopenia (bleeding, bruising and purpura).
In addition, lymphadenopathy and splenomegaly may be present and tend to be more marked in acute lymphoblastic leukaemia.
Sometimes renal and hepatic enlargement are present and there may be neurological abnormalities due to leukaemic infiltration.

272. Cosmetic or symptomatic lymphadenopathy.
Systemic symptoms due to anaemia or thrombocytopenia.
Impending or established bone marrow failure or blast transformation.
When CLL is complicated by autoimmune haemolytic anaemia.

273. Immunologically mediated reactions against red cells will lead either to:

Intravascular haemolysis with anxiety, flushing, chest or lumbar pain, tachypnoea and tachycardia followed by shock and renal failure, haemoglobin found in plasma and urine, with possible methaemalbuminaemia and reduced haptoglobin, or

Extravascular haemolysis with milder reactions than above with malaise and fever. Shock·and/or renal failure would be unlikely. Unconjugated bilirubin may rise.

In the absence of red cell destruction, most febrile reactions are due to immunity against white cells, platelets or plasma antigens.

**274.** What are the clinical features of paroxysmal nocturnal haemoglobinuria?

**275.** What are the main complications of multiple myeloma?

**276.** Mrs A. B., aged 55, complained of tiredness and epigastric pain after meals. This is her blood picture:

Hb: 6·3 g/dl                     RBC: 3·9 million/mm³
PCV: 24%                          MCV: 59 fl   MCH: 26 pg
Reticulocytes: 0·5%              Platelets: 200000/mm³
White cell count: 4800/mm³
    Differential WCC:
        Neutrophils: 49%         Lymphocytes: 44%
        Monocytes: 6%            Eosinophils: 1%
Film—hypochromia, microcytosis.

What is the likely diagnosis?

**277.** Mrs C. D., aged 45, had episodes of abdominal pain and the following blood picture:

Hb: 8·0 g/dl                     RBC: 2·3 million/mm³
PCV: 25%                          MCV: 103 fl   MCH: 30 pg
Reticulocytes: 16%              Platelets 95000/mm³
White cell count: 2900/mm³
    Differential WCC:
        Neutrophils: 60%         Lymphocytes: 35%
        Monocytes: 4%            Eosinophils: 1%
Film—occasional nucleated cells, anisocytosis, slight macrocytosis
Acid serum haemolysis test (Ham's test)— positive
Coombs' test—negative.

What is the likely diagnosis?

*Answers overleaf*

**274.** Haemoglobinuria, (although only intermittently gross), anaemia, mild granulocytopenia and thrombocytopenia, venous thrombosis in peripheral, mesenteric, hepatic, portal and cerebral veins, back pain, abdominal pain and headache.

**275.** Hypercalcaemia due to excess osteoclastic activity.
Renal failure—mainly because of tubular damage from light chains.
Infections especially with *Steptococcus pneumoniae* and herpes zoster.

**276.** Chronic iron-deficiency anaemia, possibly due to blood loss from a peptic ulcer or gastric carcinoma.

**277.** Paroxysmal nocturnal haemoglobinuria.

**278.** Mr E. F., aged 26, admitted with pneumonia, has the following picture:

| | |
|---|---|
| Hb: 8·0 g/dl | RBC: 2·1 million/mm³ |
| PCV: 24% | MCV: 120 fl   MCH: 30 pg |
| Reticulocytes: 58% | Platelets: 200000/mm³ |

White cell count: 13000/mm³
Differential WCC:

| | |
|---|---|
| Neutrophils: 70% | Lymphocytes: 23% |
| Monocytes: 6% | Eosinophils: 1% |

Film—spherocytosis, macrocytosis, polychromasia
Direct Coombs' test—positive
Ham's test—negative
Cold agglutininins—1 : 32

What is the likely diagnosis?

**279.** Mr L. T., aged 54, presented with lethargy and bleeding gums. This was his full blood count:

| | |
|---|---|
| Hb: 6·0 g/dl | RBC: 1·8 million/mm³ |
| PCV: 20% | MCV: 90 fl   MCH: 30 pg |

Platelets: 17000/mm³
White cell count: 20600/mm³
Differential WCC:

| | |
|---|---|
| Neutrophils: 14% | Lymphocytes: 5% |
| Monocytes: 5% | Promyelocytes: 11% |
| Myeloblasts: 65% | |

Film—normochromia, normocytosis

What is the diagnosis?

**280.** Mrs S. H., aged 70, consulted her G.P. because of bilateral groin swellings. Her full blood count was:

| | |
|---|---|
| Hb: 13·0 g/dl | RBC: 4·1 million/mm³ |
| PCV: 39% | MCV: 89 fl   MCH: 29 pg |

Platelets: 180000/mm³
White cell count: 175000/mm³
Differential WCC:

| | |
|---|---|
| Neutrophils: 2% | Lymphocytes: 96% |
| Monocytes: 2% | |

Film—normochromia, normocytosis

What is the diagnosis?

*Answers overleaf*

**278.** Autoimmune haemolytic anaemia due to the associated cold agglutinins of mycoplasma pneumonia.

**279.** Acute myeloblastic leukaemia.

**280.** Chronic lymphatic leukaemia.

281. Mr J. W., aged 61, a known hypertensive, is complaining of vague indigestion and headaches, A routine blood count showed:

Hb: 19 g/dl                 RBC: 7·9 million/mm³
PCV: 61%                MCV: 75 fl      MCH: 25 pg
Platelets: 680,000/mm³
White cell count: 16,000/mm³
Differential WCC:
   Neutrophils: 75%         Lymphocytes: 19%
   Monocytes: 5%            Eosinophils: 1%
Film—hypochromia, microcytosis, anisocytosis.

What is the diagnosis?

*Answers overleaf*

**281.** Polycythaemia rubra vera.

# Miscellaneous Medicine

## (Infectious Diseases, Dermatology Acid–base and Electrolyte Disorders, Genetics, Nutrition)

**282.**  What are the important serological tests for syphilis?

**283.**  List the common clinical features of secondary syphilis.

**284.**  When is syphilis most infectious?

**285.**  What is N.S.U.?

**286.**  In a suspected case of gonorrhoea, where would you swab for the organism?

**287.**  What is the treatment of choice for gonorrhoea?

*Answers overleaf*

**282.** Two types of antibody produced by the infection are the basis of the serological tests:

Nonspecific (reaginic) antibody—VDRL tests is the most commonly used and is positive in 70% of primary infections, in 100% of secondary infections, and in 70–80% of tertiary infections.

Specific antitreponemal antibody—important tests are Fluorescent Treponemal Antibody (FTA) test, Treponema Pallidum Immobilization (TPI) test and Treponema Pallidum Haemagglutination Assay (TPHA). FTA is positive in 90% of primary infections compared to 45% and 70% for TPI and TPHA; all 3 tests are 95–100% positive in the other stages.

*Note* — False positive non-specific tests occur in other diseases e.g. S.L.E.

None of these tests distinguish syphilis from other treponematoses, e.g. yaws or pinta.

**283.** Rash—usually non-pruritic, faint, dull, erythematous and macular.

Condylomata lata on perineum.

Mucous patches (or snail track ulcers) on mucous membranes of mouth.

Lymphadenopathy—generalized and painless.

**284.** Most probably during the second stage; condylomata lata are particularly infectious and contain spirochaetes.

**285.** Non-specific urethritis—most cases are probably caused by *Chlamydia trachomatis*.

**286.** In men: urethra, anal canal and rectum, and pharynx.
In women: urethra, cervix, anal canal and rectum, and pharynx.

**287.** There are 3 acceptable regimes:

Procaine penicillin 4·8 million units i.m. stat. at 2 different sites with probenecid 1 g orally.

Tetracycline 500 mg oral qds for 5 days.

Ampicillin 3·5 g (amoxycillin 3 g) oral stat. with probenecid 1 g orally.

**288.** What type of herpes virus causes genital herpes?

**289.** What type of individuals are most at risk of contracting **AIDS**?

**290.** What is the diagnostic clinical sign of measles?

**291.** Circumoral pallor and strawberry tongue are features of which infectious disease?

**292.** What disorders are caused by adenoviruses?

**293.** Compare the rash of chickenpox with that of smallpox.

*Answers overleaf*

**288.** Most cases of genital herpes are caused by herpes simplex virus type 2 but type 1 infections may be found in the genital area.

**289.** Acquired immune deficiency syndrome (AIDS) has become a very fashionable and increasingly recognized problem, particularly among male homosexuals, haemophiliacs, Haitians and heroin (or other drug) addicts. The cause is unknown but the patient usually dies, often as a result of Kaposi's sarcoma or an opportunistic infection such as pneumocystis pneumonia.

**290.** Koplik's spots—these are like grains of salt surrounded by a narrow band of inflammation and are found on the mucous membrane of the mouth. They occur in the catarrhal phase of the illness and disappear as the skin rash develops.

**291.** Scarlet fever (Scarlatina).

**292.** Upper respiratory tract infection
Febrile pharyngitis
Pharyngoconjunctival fever
Pneumonia
Pertussis-like syndrome
Keratoconjunctivitis
Acute haemorrhagic cystitis.

**293.** In chickenpox, the rash is most marked centrally, on the trunk, and the axillae are involved, whereas in smallpox, the rash is peripheral, sparing the axillae and heavily involving the forearms, forelegs and face. Chickenpox vesicles are superficial, thin-walled and fragile, elliptical and unilocular; smallpox vesicles are deep set, thick-walled, circular and multilocular. The lesions of chickenpox occur in crops so that lesions at different stages of development are seen in the same area whereas the lesions of smallpox are all at the same stage at the same time.

**294.** List the main causes of a PUO.

**295.** What is the significance of a positive Mantoux test?

**296.** What are the possible complications of influenza?

**297.** What infections cause a lymphocytosis?

**298.** What are the main clinical features of leptospirosis?

**299.** What is tertian malaria?

*Answers overleaf*

**294.** Causes of a pyrexia of unknown origin are:

Infections, e.g. T.B., subacute infective endocarditis, brucellosis, biliary infection, pyelonephritis, deep abscess.
Drugs.
Malignancy e.g. lymphoma, renal or lung carcinoma.
Connective tissue disease.

**295.** It shows that the patient has delayed hypersensitivity to tubercle bacilli as a result of active infection, previous infection or B.C.G. vaccination.

**296.** Tracheitis, bronchitis
Pneumonia—primary viral
           secondary bacterial (much commoner than viral type)
Cardiomyopathy
Encephalitis.

**297.** Pertussis, infectious hepatitis, T.B., brucellosis, syphilis, benign infectious lymphocytosis, infectious mononucleosis (atypical lymphocytes).

**298.** Relevant occupational or exposure history
Fever, headache
Petechial haemorrhages
Jaundice (because of hepatitis)
Meningism (because of mengingitis)
Tachycardia, hypotension, cardiomegaly (because of myocarditis)
Acute renal failure (because of tubular necrosis).

**299.** This is the characteristic malaria of *Plasmodium vivax* or *Plasmodium ovale* infections; the fever returns regularly on every third day after the first week of the illness during which the fever is erratic.

**300.** Which is potentially the most serious form of malaria?

**301.** What malaria prophylaxis would you recommend to a person travelling to an endemic area?

**302.** What is the treatment of choice for typhoid fever?

**303.** What infections are associated with peripheral blood eosinophilia?

**304.** How would you treat amoebic dysentery?

**305.** Do you know of any drugs which can cause photosensitivity?

*Answers overleaf*

**300.** *Plasmodium falciparum* malaria; it can cause cerebral malaria or blackwater fever (intravascular haemolysis) both of which may be fatal.

**301.** Chloroquine 500 mg weekly to be continued 6 weeks after return from the endemic area. If the area is known to have chloroquine-resistant strains, pyrimethamine and sulfadoxine should be taken in addition to chloroquine. Chloroquine eradicates *P. malariae* and *P. falciparum; P. vivax* and *P. ovale* will only be suppressed by it, therefore patient may need a course of primaquine after cessation of chloroquine therapy.

**302.** Chloramphenicol; ampicillin or co-trimoxazole may be used as alternatives but they are neither as predictable nor as effective as chloramphenicol.

**303.** Eosinophilia is only seen in patients with parasitic, especially helminthic, infections.

**304.** General measures—replace fluid losses and provide symptomatic treatment for the diarrhoea.
Specific measures—in a mild to moderate attack, metronidazole with diiodohydroxyquin or diloxanide furoate; in a severe attack, add emetine or dehydroemetine to the above regime. If the patient has extra-intestinal involvement (e.g. liver abscess), treat with either metronidazole or chloroquine plus emetine.

**305.** Systemic drugs: sulphonamides
sulphonylureas
thiazides
frusemide
tetracyclines
phenothiazines
nalidixic acid
chlordiazepoxide
oral contraceptives
Topical drugs: hexachlorophane
para-aminobenzoic acid
coal tar derivatives

**306.** What are the possible causes of erythema nodosum?

**307.** What might cause generalized pruritus without diagnostic skin lesions?

**308.** Of what disease is lupus pernio a cutaneous manifestation?

**309.** Do you know of any skin disorders that may indicate internal malignancy?

**310.** What skin lesions may be seen in diabetics?

*Answers overleaf*

**306.** Sarcoidosis
Group B haemolytic streptococcal infections
Tuberculosis
Inflammatory bowel disease (ulcerative colitis; Crohn's disease)
Drugs, e.g. penicillin, sulphonamides, bromides, iodides, some oral
contraceptives
Yersiniosis
Systemic fungal infections, e.g. histoplasmosis
Leprosy

**307.** Psychogenic states
Dry skin
'Senile' pruritus
Biliary obstruction, especially primary biliary cirrhosis
Polycythaemia rubra vera
Lymphoma and leukaemia
Chronic renal failure
Skin infestations
Opiate drugs

**308.** Sarcoidosis; it is a nodular or plaque-like lesion of dark violet colour
which most characteristially affects the tip of the nose.
Considerable swelling and disfigurement may occur.

**309.** Dermatomyositis
Acanthosis nigricans
Migratory thrombophlebitis
Icthyosis
Tylosis palmaris.

**310.** Lesions associated with diabetes mellitus:
Necrobiosis lipoidica diabeticorum
Granuloma annulare
Diabetic dermopathy (spotted leg syndrome)

Lesions related to hyperglycaemia and glycosuria:
Boils and carbuncles
Candidiasis of the vulva, glans penis or surrounding skin.

Lesions caused by complications of diabetes:
Ulceration
Gangrene.

**311.** What is mycosis fungoides?

**312.** What endocrine disorders may be associated with mucocutaneous candidiasis?

**313.** What skin disorders can be associated with ulcerative colitis or Crohn's disease?

**314.** What are Campbell de Morgan spots?

**315.** What is the significance of vitiligo?

**316.** Do you know what might cause attacks of facial flushing?

**317.** What disorders may be associated with a malar flush?

**318.** What is von Recklinghausen's disease of the skin better known as?

*Answers overleaf*

**311.** A primary T-cell lymphoma of the skin; it may be preceded by many years of non-specific eczematous or psoriaform lesions.

**312.** Hypoparathyroidism
Hypothyroidism
Adrenal insufficiency
Diabetes mellitus.

**313.** Erythema nodosum
Pyoderma gangrenosum.

**314.** Small haemangiomatous lesions, red in colour, about 1–2 mm in diameter and standing above the skin surface, which are commonly seen in older people. They have no clinical significance.

**315.** Vitiligo is an acquired circumscribed patchy or generalized loss of pigmentation of the skin; it may be familial and commonly is of no significance. However in patients over 50, it may be associated with autoimmune and endocrine disorders, e.g. pernicious anaemia, Addison's disease, diabetes mellitus, hypothyroidism and other thyroid disorders.

**316.** Menopause
Drugs e.g. nitrates
chlorpropamide (with alcohol)
metronidazole (with alcohol)
Alcohol
Carcinoid syndrome and VIPoma are very rare causes.

**317.** Mitral stenosis
Hypothyroidism.

**318.** Neurofibromatosis.

**319.** What is erythema ab igne?

**320.** Trisomy 21 is the genetic nomenclature for what condition and what are the clinical features?

**321.** What is the sex chromosome constitution of Turner's syndrome and Klinefelter's syndrome?

**322.** What is the risk of a child of two parents heterozygous for a recessive condition being affected?

**323.** What is the mode of inheritance of classic haemophilia and how are the children of a woman who carries the trait and a normal man affected?

**324.** What is the anion gap?

*Answers overleaf*

**319.** Also known as 'Granny's tartan', it is a form of livedo reticularis seen in areas of the skin to which heat has often been applied. There is a persistent red or brown discoloration of the skin in a characteristic fishnet pattern. The commonest site is the forelegs of elderly patients who sit too near a fire.

**320.** Down's syndrome or mongolism.
The clinical features include widely spaced (hypertelorism) and upward slanting eyes, epicanthic folds, malformed ears, broad or short neck and single transverse palmar crease. There is mental retardation, and an increased frequency of associated conditions such as congenital heart disease, acute leukaemia and duodenal atresia.

**321.** XO is the commonest configuration for Turner's syndrome although mosaics and other forms are seen.
XXY is the commonest configuration for affected males with Klinefelter's syndrome but up to 4 X chromosomes may be present. XXYY is sometimes seen.

**322.** 1 in 4.

**323.** Haemophilia is an X-linked recessive condition. Half the sons will carry the affected gene and therefore have the condition because, although recessive, it is unopposed by a normal X chromosome.
Half the daughters will also carry the gene but will not be affected because of the recessive nature of the X-linked gene.

**324.** It is a derived figure obtained by subtracting the sum of plasma bicarbonate and chloride from the sum of plasma sodium and potassium concentration.
It is elevated in cases of acidosis not due to loss of bicarbonate or administration of chloride. It may be a pointer to the presence of lactic acidosis when no other cause for metabolic acidosis is obvious.

**325.** List some causes of metabolic acidosis.

**326.** What is hyponatraemia and how would you classify it?

**327.** What are the clinical features of hypernatraemia?

**328.** What are the E.C.G. abnormalities of hypokalaemia?

**329.** What conditions are associated with, and what are the clinical features of, magnesium deficiency?

*Answers overleaf*

**325.** The causes can be grouped under three headings:
Increased production of acid
e.g. diabetic ketoacidosis
lactic acidosis secondary to shock or certain drugs, e.g. phenformin
Decreased acid excretion by the kidney, e.g. chronic renal failure, renal tubular acidosis.
Loss of bicarbonate e.g. diarrhoea.

**326.** It is the finding of a plasma sodium concentration below normal and can be classified into:
True sodium depletion (i.e. volume depletion) requiring the replacement of salt and water.
Dilutional hyponatraemia where the total body sodium is normal but excess water dilutes plasma sodium. Restriction of water intake may be necessary.
An incompletely understood category of essential hyponatraemia or 'sick cell syndrome' where, usually in the context of severe illness, there is a leaking of water out of cells diluting the plasma sodium.

**327.** There are two types of hypernatraemia:
A pure water deficit which results in intracellular dehydration and confusion progressing to stupor and coma.
A deficit of both sodium and water which causes signs of extracellular volume depletion, i.e. dry mucous membranes, decreased skin turgor, postural hypotension, reduced intraocular pressure, lethargy and weakness.

**328.** Flattening or inversion of the T wave
Increased prominence of the U wave
Sagging of the ST segments.

**329.** Chronic diarrhoea and malnutrition especially in the 'short bowel syndrome', prolonged diarrhoea and vomiting. Clinical features are mainly neuromuscular irritability with tremor, choreiform movements and tetany usually in association with hypocalcaemia.

**330.** What tests or clinical measurements would you perform to determine the presence of generalized malnutrition?

**331.** What is anorexia nervosa?

**332.** In addition to minerals, vitamins and electrolytes, what solutions are administered during parenteral nutrition?

**333.** What are the clinical features of vitamin A deficiency?

**334.** What diseases does obesity predispose to?

**335.** Briefly describe Wernicke's encephalopathy and Korsakoff's psychosis. In what sort of patients do these conditions occur?

*Answers overleaf*

**330.** Body weight—expressed as a percentage of known previous healthy weight.

Triceps skinfold thickness (TSF) (measured with callipers) and arm muscle circumference (determined from measuring arm circumference and TSF), both expressed as a percentage of standard.

Plasma proteins, particularly albumin, transferrin, retinol binding protein and pre-albumin.

Immunological tests—particularly total lymphocyte count or delayed hypersensitivity response to skin testing.

**331.** It is a disorder of previously healthy adolescent girls who become emaciated as a result of voluntary starvation.

**332.** Amino acid solutions—usually synthetic.

Glucose solutions—or other carbohydrate energy source although glucose is to be preferred.

Fat solutions usually soya bean oil emulsion—both to provide essential fatty acid requirements and as a calorie source.

**333.** Night blindness, xerosis (dryness of the conjunctiva)

Bitot's spots (small grey plaques on conjunctiva)

Keratomalacia with ulceration and necrosis of the cornea.

The end result is blindness.

**334.** Osteoarthritis, especially of hips, knees and spine

Abdominal hernia, hiatal hernia

Hyperlipidaemia, gallstones, hyperuricaemia

Non-insulin dependent diabetes mellitus

Hypertension.

**335.** Wernicke's encephalopathy is manifest by ocular disturbance, usually some form of bilateral symmetrical ophthalmoplegia accompanied by both horizontal and vertical nystagmus. Cerebellar ataxia and cranial nerve palsies are frequently present.

Korsakoff's psychosis is a defect in retentive memory and learning characterized by confabulation, and can be regarded as the psychic component of Wernicke's disease.

The aetiology of these conditions is thiamine deficiency. Although cases are occasionally seen in simple nutritonal deficiency, the majority of patients are alcoholics.

# Neurology

**336.** What organisms commonly cause bacterial meningitis in adults?

**337.** If an adult patient with bacterial meningitis is too ill to wait for C.S.F. bacteriology, how would you treat him?

**338.** What changes in the C.S.F. would you expect in tuberculous meningitis?

**339.** What are the possible sequelae of bacterial meningitis?

**340.** What is the most important complication of trigeminal herpes zoster infection?

**341.** Does poliomyelitis cause sensory loss?

*Answers overleaf*

**336.** *Neisseria meningitidis* (meningococcus)—50%
*Haemophilus influenzae* ⎫
*Streptococcus pneumoniae* ⎬ —30–40%

**337.** If the patient is too ill to wait for the gram stain result or, more usually, the result is inconclusive, treatment should be started at once although the choice of antibiotics to be given is controversial. As meningococcus, haemophilus or pneumococcus are the most likely causes, probably the wisest choice is parenteral chloramphenicol and benzyl-penicillin. A few physicians would still add sulphadimidine to this combination. Others would use ampicillin and chloramphenicol in combination.

**338.** Protein moderately or greatly elevated
Sugar greatly depressed or absent
Lymphocytosis with or without neutrophilia
Clear fluid with 'cobweb' clot after standing
Organisms on gram stain, after guinea pig inoculation, and on culture.

**339.** Deafness
Cranial nerve palsies
Hemiplegia
Hydrocephalus
Epilepsy
Dementia
Sequelae are much more common with haemophilus and pneumococcus than meningococcus

**340.** Corneal ulceration as a result of involvement of the ophthalmic branch of the trigeminal nerve.

**341.** No—poliomyelitis only affects anterior horn cells so causes lower motor neurone signs.

**342.** List some of the causes of cerebral haemorrhage.

**343.** What are the signs of subarachnoid haemorrhage?

**344.** What are poor diagnostic signs in subarachnoid harmorrhage?

**345.** What are the major signs of internal capsule haemorrhage?

*Answers overleaf*

**342.** Hypertension
Atheroma
Haemorrhagic infarct
Aneurysm—congenital, mycotic
Angioma and other tumour
Coagulopathy
Trauma
Unknown

**343.** Disordered consciousness—often coma
Pyrexia
Meningeal irritation
Retinal, subhyaloid or vitreous haemorrhages
Depressed or absent tendon and abdominal reflexes with extensor
    plantars (usually rapidly recover and do not necessarily mean
    focal neurological damage).
Albuminuria and glycosuria
Focal signs only appear if there has been intracerebral extension of
    the haemorrhage.

**344.** Increasing depth of coma
Rising pulse and respiratory rate
Increasing fever
Evidence of cerebral hemisphere extension
No sign of recovery in 48 h.

**345.** Coma
Slow bounding pulse
Deep and stertorous respiration
Head and eyes deviated to side of bleed
Upper motor neurone facial palsy on opposite side from bleed
Hemiplegia on opposite side from bleed
Hemianaesthesia on paralysed side
Initial absence of reflexes and depressed tone ('neuronal shock')

**346.**  What are transient cerebral ischaemic attacks?

**347.**  How would you manage transient cerebral ischaemic attacks?

**348.**  List some of the causes of cerebral embolus.

**349.**  How would you diagnose a chronic subdural haematoma?

*Answers overleaf*

**346.** Recurrent neurological episodes following ischaemia to an area of the brain supplied by the carotid arteries or vertebrobasilar system. They may last for a few seconds or up to 12 h with complete recovery between attacks. The neurological signs may be the same during each attack or may be different. Platelet emboli from atheromatous plaques especially in a stenosed carotid artery are frequently blamed. They are important because they often precede an established stroke.

**347.** Long-term anticoagulants or antiplatelet drugs (e.g. aspirin, dipyridamole) may stop attacks and prevent a completed stroke. Surgery should be considered in patients with arterial obstruction in the subclavian or carotid arteries. If surgery is not feasible anticoagulants or antiplatelet drugs are indicated in frequent or severe attacks, in attacks of long duration or in attacks which fail to clear completely. Anticoagulants may be replaced by antiplatelet drugs after 3–6 months. The patient should stop smoking. There is no evidence that cerebral vasodilators are of any value. Two-thirds of patients have hypertension which should be carefully treated as an abrupt fall in blood pressure may precipitate a completed stroke.

**348.** Atrial fibrillation, especially if an attempt has been made to convert longstanding atrial fibrillation to sinus rhythm.
Mitral stenosis with or without atrial fibrillation
Myocardial infarction
Atheroma, especially in carotid and subclavian arteries
Cardiac surgery
Infective endocarditis

Rarer causes—tumour embolus, septic embolus (from lung abscess), fat embolus (long bone fracture), paradoxical embolus, atrial myxoma.

**349.** The diagnosis may be suggested by the clinical features and pineal shift on skull X-ray but is confirmed by CT scan. If CT scans are not available, exploratory burr holes will be necessary if the diagnosis is suspected.

**350.** In what sort of patient should you consider the diagnosis of chronic subdural haematoma?

**351.** How would you manage a patient with a subarachnoid haemorrhage?

**352.** When are anticoagulants indicated in patients with cerebrovascular accidents?

**353.** Are upper or lower motor neurones involved in motor neurone disease?

**354.** What C.S.F. changes may be found in multiple sclerosis?

*Answers overleaf*

350. **In the elderly.** They frequently have no recollection of any head injury and present with non-specific symptoms such as headache, confusion, giddiness, mental slowing and, rarely, fits. There is rarely evidence of focal neurological damage although hemiplegia or aphasia may be found. Ipsilateral pupillary dilatation and ptosis with coma are very late signs.

351. General measures:
    Absolute bed rest 4–8 weeks
    Head of bed raised
    Straining at stool avoided by laxatives
    Anticonvulsants given if necessary
    Hypertension, if present, is treated carefully

    Localization of bleeding site:
    Carotid and vertebral angiography (positive in 85%) when situation has stabilized

    Prevention of rebleeding:
    Epsiaminocaproic acid 24 g/day for three weeks is increasingly being used to impede clot lysis at the site of the ruptured aneurysm.
    Surgery is undertaken 1–2 weeks after the bleed if the site of bleeding has been visualized and is accessible.

352. **In cerebral embolism and in transient cerebral ischaemic attacks.** There is no evidence that they are beneficial in completed stroke due to cerebral thrombosis. They are contraindicated in cerebral haemorrhage. Before anticoagulating a stroke patient, a CT scan is mandatory to exclude cerebral haemorrhage.

353. **Both.** Anterior horn cells and anterior nerve roots of the cord degenerate to cause lower motor neurone signs and direct and crossed corticospinal tracts degenerate leading to upper motor neurone signs. Many patients have both upper and lower motor neurone signs.

354. C.S.F. abnormalities are found in 50% of cases. Possible findings are an excess of mononuclear cells, abnormal colloidal gold curve (usually paretic, occasionally luetic), elevated IgG with or without an increase in total protein.

**355.** What features of multiple sclerosis are associated with a poor prognosis?

**356.** How would you treat multiple sclerosis?

**357.** What are the causes of a lower motor neurone facial palsy?

**358.** What are the clinical differences between an upper and a lower motor neurone facial palsy?

**359.** List some of the signs of dystrophia myotonica.

*Answers overleaf*

**355.** Failure to remit completely after first attack, a short initial remission, or insidious onset.

**356.** Many and varied treatments have been proposed and tried such as gluten free diet, sunflower oil (linoleic acid), but there is no satisfactory treatment of the disease. ACTH is of value in treating acute exacerbations but many patients fail to show any response to it. Management involves explanation, understanding, support, counselling, physiotherapy and specific help for problems such as pressure sores, urinary retention and spasticity.

**357.** Bell's palsy
Surgery (especially to parotid gland)
Basal skull fracture
Pontine haemorrhage
Acoustic neuroma
Pontine tumour
Tumour involving temporal lobe
Geniculate ganglion herpes zoster (Ramsay Hunt syndrome)
Sarcoidosis

**358.** In the lower motor neurone palsy, muscles of the upper and lower part of the face are equally involved. In the upper motor neurone palsy, the muscles of the upper face (frontalis and orbicularis oculis) are less affected because of the bilateral upper motor neurone innervation to that part of the face. Moreover in an upper motor neurone lesion, the weakness of the lower face apparent on voluntary movement may disappear during emotional facial movement.

**359.** Myotonia
Muscle atrophy (especially temporalis and sternomastoids)
Distal muscle weakness (an exception to the rule that myopathic weakness is more marked proximally)
Mask-like facies with ptosis
Frontal baldness
Testicular atrophy
Cataracts
Reduced tendon jerks
Mental retardation and dementia.

**360.** What is Friedreich's ataxia?

**361.** Can migraine cause hemiplegia?

**362.** What are the causes of ptosis?

**363.** What are the commonest causes of headache?

**364.** List the types of involuntary movements you know.

*Answers overleaf*

**360.** It is a progressive disorder with degeneration of the cerebellum, spinocerebellar tracts, pyramidal tracts, dorsal columns, and peripheral nerves. It is inherited usually as an autosomal recessive. Typical cases have cerebellar ataxia, severe limb weaknesses, kyphoscoliosis (for reasons that are uncertain), pes cavus, cocking of the toes, absent tendon jerks and extensor plantars (an unusual combination), loss of vibration and joint position sense and some evidence of symmetrical loss of light touch, pain and temperature sensation in the limbs. ECG changes may occur and death occurs in early adult life, often from cardiomyopathy.

**361.** Probably yes, but if it occurs, it is rare and usually transitory. If a patient presents with migraine and hemiplegia, an underlying arteriovenous malformation or other cause should be considered before ascribing the hemiplegia to migraine, especially in the elderly who may be getting transient cerebral ischaemic attacks.

**362.** Third nerve palsy
Sympathetic fibre destruction (e.g. Horner's syndrome)
Myopathy (dystrophia myotonica, myasthenia gravis)
Other (congenital, hysterical).

**363.** Migraine and tension headaches—90% of cases presenting to a doctor.

**364.** Tremor
Tic
Chorea
Athetosis
Hemiballismus
Dystonia
Myoclonus

**365.** What are the clinical features of raised intracranial pressure?

**366.** What are the signs of an upper motor neurone lesion?

**367.** What are the signs of a lower motor neurone lesion?

**368.** What is meant by the term 'mononeuritis multiplex'?

**369.** What are the signs of a cerebellar lesion?

*Answers overleaf*

**365.** Early:
　　Headache—unilateral or diffuse; throbbing or bursting
　　Vomiting—projectile without nausea
　　Papilloedema and visual failure.
　Late:
　　Progressive drowsiness to coma
　　Fits
　　False localizing signs, e.g. 3rd or 6th nerve palsies, bilateral
　　　extensor plantars.
　Very late:
　　Fixed dilated pupils
　　Deep coma

**366.** Weakness or paralysis of movements
　Increased tone
　Increased reflexes, sometimes accompanied by clonus
　An extensor plantar response.

**367.** Weakness or paralysis of muscles
　Reduced tone
　Diminished reflexes. Normal plantar response, unless damage to
　　peripheral nerves governing movements of great toe
　Wasting of the affected muscles
　Fasciculation may be present.

**368.** Mononeuritis multiplex is the term given to involvement of two or
　more peripheral nerves, with clinical signs limited to discrete
　neural territories and occurs in such conditions as polyarteritis
　nodosa, diabetes mellitus, sarcoidosis.

**369.** Ipsilateral:
　　Reduced tone
　　Diminished or pendular reflexes
　　Ataxic gait often tending towards the side of the lesion
　　Disorders of movement including:
　　　past pointing
　　　intention tremor
　　　dysdiadochokinesis—which is failure to perform rapid
　　　　alternating movements such as pronation and supination of
　　　　hand.
　Sometimes scanning speech and nystagmus are present.

**370.** Where is the site of the lesion which causes a right upper homonomous quadrantanopia?

**371.** What are features of a parietal lobe lesion?

**372.** What investigations may be carried out on a specimen of C.S.F.?

**373.** What further information is obtained during actual performance of lumbar puncture?

**374.** Describe the fundal manifestation of papilloedema.

*Answers overleaf*

**370.** In the optic radiation of the left temporal lobe.

**371.** Sensory epilepsy
Apraxia—inability to perform a complex action in the absence of motor or sensory deficit
Agnosia—inability to recognize a familiar object
Sensory inattention
Receptive dysphasia
Homonymous hemi- or quadrantanopia.

**372.** Inspection for:
Blood in three separate specimens
Xanthochromia after spinning
Clarity; cloudiness denotes meningitis
Clot formation as in tuberculous meningitis
Microscopy for:
Cell count
Organisms after gram staining
Biochemistry for:
Total protein
Immunoglobulins
Glucose
Culture
Serology, particularly for syphilis and viruses.

**373.** Whether the tap is clean or traumatic—take 3 specimens
The C.S.F. pressure—normal is 50–150 mm $H_2O$
The presence of free rise and fall with respiration
Queckenstedt's test. Compression of the jugular veins in the neck normally causes an increase in the pressure of C.S.F., and this may be absent in a block of the spinal canal.

**374.** Engorgement of retinal veins
Pink colouration of optic disc
Blurring of disc margins
Swelling of disc with obliteration of physiological cup
Retinal haemorrhages may be present.

**375.** What may cause a similar appearance to papilloedema?

**376.** Classify the causes of optic atrophy.

**377.** How is/are the paretic muscle(s) identified in a patient with diplopia due to a paretic squint?

**378.** What are the two most common causes of vertigo in a young man?

**379.** How would you treat a patient with trigeminal neuralgia?

*Answers overleaf*

**375.** Optic neuritis with involvement of the optic nerve head, for example due to multiple sclerosis, or rarer causes such as syphilis, methyl alcohol toxicity or vitamin $B_{12}$ deficiency. Differentiation from papilloedema is made on the almost complete preservation of visual fields in papilloedema, but a significant central scotoma with loss of vision in optic neuritis.

**376.** Primary—direct damage to the optic nerve head:
Pressure on optic nerve by a space-occupying lesion
Following head injury involving frontal region or orbit
Following retrobulbar neuritis, multiple sclerosis or syphilis
Following vascular occlusive lesions of optic nerve in arteriosclerosis, diabetes, cranial arteritis, obstruction of central artery of retina (e.g. embolic)
Toxins: methyl alcohol, tobacco, quinine.
Secondary to papilloedema. Disc margin remains blurred.
Consecutive upon conditions of the retina or eye such as choroidoretinitis, glaucoma, retinitis pigmentosa.

**377.** The direction of gaze producing the greatest separation of images is identified. The most peripheral image, identified by covering one eye and then the other, is produced by the affected eye. The muscle(s) responsible for that direction of gaze is paretic.

**378.** Vestibular neuritis which is characterized by the abrupt onset of vertigo, nausea and vomiting, without the impairment of hearing. The attacks are brief and often leave the patient with mild positional vertigo for some days. The cause is unknown.
Multiple sclerosis. Nystagmus and vertigo are common presenting features of this condition in young adults.

**379.** Treatment is frequently unsatisfactory but relief may be obtained using carbamazepine, phenytoin or clonazepam.
Phenol block by injection into the Gasserian ganglion produces facial hemianaesthesia, and interrupts corneal sensation.
Section of the sensory component of the 5th nerve requires intracranial operation, but corneal sensation may be preserved.

**380.** What are the clinical features of Bell's palsy?

**381.** A 50-year-old man presents with recurrent paroxysms of vertigo associated with tinnitus and progressive nerve deafness. What is the likely diagnosis?

**382.** How would you investigate a 43-year-old woman who presented with a recent history of two grand mal seizures?

**383.** What percentage of intracranial tumours are meningiomas and why is their specific diagnosis important?

**384.** What are the features of classic migraine?

*Answers overleaf*

**380.** A prodromal symptom of ache near the angle of the jaw is followed between a few hours and 2 days by unilateral lower motor neurone facial paralysis. In a minority of cases there is loss of taste on the anterior two-thirds of tongue, and hyperacusis, due to involvement of the nerve to stapedius.

**381.** Menière's syndrome. This is suggested by the paroxysmal nature of the episodes, although other causes of the symptoms, particularly acoustic neuroma, should be excluded.

**382.** Confirm that the seizures are epileptiform by:
Direct observation—rarely possible
Interviewing witness
Careful history of prodromata and sequelae from patient
EEG—can be helpful but a normal EEG does not exclude epilepsy.
Exclude metabolic causes, e.g. hypoglycaemia and cardiac causes.
Exclude a structural abnormality, particularly space-occupying lesion by:
EEG
Skull radiology
CT scan of brain

**383.** Approximately 20% of intracranial tumours are meningiomas. Their specific diagnosis is important because they are almost always benign, encapsulated and completely removable.

**384.** Classic migraine is characterized by some or all of the following features:
Vague premonition of impending attack.
Visual disturbance consisting of bright lights, zig-zag lines, or fortification spectra, and scotomatous defects.
Numbness and tingling of lips, face, hands.
Mild dysphasia.
Recession of the above followed by severe throbbing unilateral headache, which lasts hours or even up to two days.
Nausea and vomiting associated with the peak of the headache.

**385.** Describe how you would treat a 25-year-old man who experienced frequent attacks of migraine.

**386.** What is the differential diagnosis of nuchal (neck) rigidity?

**387.** What is the prognosis of subarachnoid haemorrhage?

**388.** What are the clinical features of a severe pontine haemorrhage?

*Answers overleaf*

**385.** Prophylaxis should be considered when the frequency of attacks is disrupting the daily life of the patient. The following drugs may be tried, but are variably successful:

Diazepam

Clonidine—in small dosage—may aggravate depression and cause insomnia

Pizotifen—causes weight gain

Methysergide—the risk of retroperitoneal and heart valve fibrosis limits its use

Propranolol—is effective in 60% patients but is limited by the usual contraindications and by interaction with ergotamine.

Treatment of the attack: Simple analgesics such as paracetamol may be sufficient. Improved absorption can be accomplished by stimulating gastric emptying with metoclopramide. Ergotamine acts by constricting cranial arteries, but side effects such as vomiting, abdominal pain, muscular cramp and habituation limit its use. It should not be repeated at intervals of less than 4 days because of risk of ergotism with gangrene.

**386.** Subarachnoid haemorrhage

Meningitis (including viral)

Meningism—neck stiffness associated with acute specific fevers, otitis media and pneumonia in childhood

Cervical spondylosis—may cause some articular stiffness but this can be differentiated from muscular spasm.

**387.** Approximately 50% will die from the existing or future subarachnoid haemorrhage, 15% within 48 h, 25% between 2 days and 6 weeks and 10% after 6 weeks. Of the survivors 10% will have severe impairment. The maximum risk of rebleeding is in the second week after the initial event.

**388.** Deep coma is usually present. There is total paralysis, decerebrate rigidity (clenched jaw, retracted neck, arms and legs stiffly extended and internally rotated) and small, pinpoint pupils. Terminal hyperpyrexia is common.

**389.** Give the headings under which you would write an essay on the management of stroke.

**390.** Describe the main ways in which multiple sclerosis presents.

*Answers overleaf*

**389.** General measures:

Care of unconscious patient
Maintenance of fluid and nutritional balance
Prevention of pressure sores by appropriate nursing measures, and possible urinary catheterization
Commencement of passive physiotherapy

Specific measures:

Confirmation of diagnosis—if cerebrovascular disease is not likely, consider further investigation with CT scan etc.
Specific treatment of meningovascular syphilis, subdural haematoma, subarachnoid haemorrhage, etc.
Possible use of dextran, especially for stroke in evolution or in young patients
Dexamethasone—where cerebral oedema is a factor
Evacuation of any developing clot surgically.

Rehabilitation:

Physiotherapy
Speech therapy
Use of aids
Modification of home
Occupational therapy.

Prevention of recurrence:

Anticoagulants for definite cerebral emboli
Treatment of hypertension.

**390.** 40% per cent have an episode of optic neuritis as their initial symptom with partial or total loss of vision in one eye often accompanied by pain or movement on the eye. Other presentations include tingling of the extremities due to posterior column involvement, or weakness of one or more limbs. Diplopia as a result of brainstem lesions, nystagmus, vertigo and cerebellar ataxia are also common presentations.

**391.** What, in general terms, are the features which enable a diagnosis of multiple sclerosis to be made?

**392.** What are the causes of Parkinsonism?

*Answers overleaf*

**391.** No single feature or laboratory test is pathognomonic. Evidence of dissemination in both time and site of lesion is required before the diagnosis can be made. Thus although the diagnosis can be suspected after a single episode of demyelination, a history of relapse and remission and signs indicating multiple lesions are required before the diagnosis can be confirmed. Even so, conditions such as spinal cord compression, neurosyphilis and sometimes vitamin $B_{12}$ deficiency may need to be excluded. A finding of increased IgG in the CSF is further evidence of M.S.

**392.** Idiopathic (paralysis agitans)—
due to damage to interconnecting system between substantia nigra and corpus striatum.

Post-encephalitis—especially as a late sequela of encephalitis lethargica, and occasionally other encephalitides.

Drugs: phenothiazines
butyrophenones such as haloperidol
reserpine
$\alpha$-methyl dopa

Infrequent causes include cerebral tumours, meningovascular syphilis, manganese and carbon monoxide poisoning, and Wilson's disease.

N.B. Atherosclerosis is no longer considered to be a cause of Parkinsonism.

**393.** What drugs are used in the treatment of Parkinson's disease?

**394.** What is the differential diagnosis of lower motor neurone lesions in the arms with sensory symptoms, and upper motor neurone lesions in the legs?

**395.** Outline the clinical features of subacute combined degeneration of the cord.

**393.** L-dopa is very effective, especially in relieving hypokinesis.

It is best given combined with a dopadecarboxylase inhibitor which reduces the amount of L-dopa required for a therapeutic effect and also diminishes the side effects, such as nausea, vomiting and cardiac arrhythmias.

Anticholinergic drugs e.g. benzhexol, benztropine, orphenadrine are no longer drugs of first choice but they still have a part to play in those 20% patients who do not respond to L-dopa, or in whom side effects of L-dopa are disabling. Side effects of anticholinergics include dryness of mouth, blurred vision, and also confusion and hallucination in the elderly.

Bromocriptine, a dopamine agonist, is also useful but should not be used as a first-line drug.

Amantidine, an antiviral agent, has anti-Parkinsonian effects and can be given with L-dopa.

**394.** To account for these features by one lesion, the site must be the cervical cord and possibilities include:
Cervical spondylosis with osteophytes compressing spinal cord
Rheumatoid arthritis with vertebral subluxation
Multiple sclerosis
Syringomyelia
Spinal cord tumours.

**395.** Paraesthesiae of toes and fingers due to peripheral neuropathy.
Difficulty holding small objects.
Weakness and ataxia which appear early but become severe later.
Signs include 'objective' sensory loss in glove and stocking distribution, impairment of vibration and position sense with sensory ataxia, absent ankle jerks (though occasionally these are increased if lateral columns are involved and peripheral nerves are intact).

**396.** Differentiate between chorea, athetosis and hemiballismus.

**397.** What are the 3 main clinical patterns of motor neurone disease?

**398.** Outline the treatment of myasthenia gravis.

*Answers overleaf*

**396.** Chorea (from the Greek for 'dance')—forcible rapid jerky movements which are involuntary but may be combined into voluntary movements as if in an attempt to make them less noticeable; they are irregular, quick and of brief duration.

Athetosis (from the Greek for 'changeable')—slow sinuous writhing and purposeless movements; they are slower than chorea but features of both can be seen in the same patient (choreoathetosis).

Hemiballismus—wild flailing movements of wide amplitude; they are much more violent than chorea.

**397.** Amyotrophic lateral sclerosis is the commonest presentation and is characterized by lower motor neurone signs in the arms and upper motor neurone signs in the legs; The prognosis is 4–5 years.

Progressive bulbar palsy is characterized by dysarthria, dysphonia and dysphagia. Wasting and fasciculation of the tongue is accompanied by a brisk jaw jerk; Death usually results from pneumonia and respiratory failure within 2 years of the onset.

Progressive muscular atrophy is characterized by lower motor neurone lesions in the legs and arms; This has the best prognosis with death in 8–10 years from the onset.

**398.** Anticholinesterase drugs, e.g. neostigmine, pyridostigmine; cumulative effects of long-acting preparations may result in cholinergic block.

Thymectomy—always performed if there is a thymoma.

High dose steroids.

Plasmapheresis may be helpful where other measures have failed.

**399.** List some of the causes of peripheral neuropathy.

**400.** What are restrictions on driving for someone with epilepsy?

*Answers overleaf*

**399.** Important causes are:

Toxins, e.g. lead, arsenic

Drugs, e.g. nitrofurantoin, isoniazid, vincristine, metronidazole.

Deficiency states and metabolic disorders, e.g. chronic alcoholism, beri-beri, pellagra, subacute combined degeneration, carcinoma of the lung, diabetes mellitus, porphyria, amyloidosis, uraemia.

Inflammatory states, e.g. Guillain-Barré syndrome, sarcoidosis, leprosy.

Vascular disease, e.g. polyarteritis nodosa, rheumatoid arthritis, diabetes mellitus.

Miscellaneous—idiopathic, genetically determined.

**400.** To hold a driving licence a person suffering from epilepsy must have been free from any attack for 2 years. However, patients with attacks only during sleep may hold a driving licence provided that they have had no other types of epileptic attacks for at least 3 years.

# Renal Medicine

**401.** List the organisms which commonly cause acute pyelonephritis.

**402.** What factors predispose to attacks of acute urinary tract infection?

**403.** How would you confirm the diagnosis of renal tuberculosis?

**404.** What is the significance of a raised serum creatinine?

*Answers overleaf*

**401.** *E. coli* (causes 90% of acute infections in patients without urological abnormalities or calculi).

Proteus, Klebsiella, Enterobacter, Serratia, Pseudomonas (commoner causes of infection in patients with recurrent infection, calculi, indwelling catheter, urological abnormalities and after urological surgery).

*Streptococcus faecalis, Staphylococcus aureus.*

**402.** Female sex
Pregnancy
Urinary obstruction
Neurogenic bladder
Vesico-ureteric reflux
Developmental anomalies of urinary tract
Renal disease and hypertension
Diabetes mellitus.

**403.** The diagnosis is suggested by painless haematuria (gross or microscopic) or by 'sterile' pyuria. Diagnosis is confirmed by finding *M. tuberculosis* in early morning urine specimens. The extent of disease is shown by I.V.P. Cystoscopy and retrograde pyelography may be necessary in extensive disease.

**404.** It suggests impaired glomerular filtration. Creatinine is endogenously produced from muscle metabolism and is not absorbed or excreted by renal tubules. It is a better indicator of renal failure than blood urea which is affected by blood volume changes and by liver disease. Creatinine clearance measurement gives a value for the glomerular filtration rate.

**405.** What does uncontrolled high blood pressure do to kidneys?

**406.** When may a palpable kidney be found?

**407.** Does a renal artery bruit have any significance?

**408.** What are the main indications for renal dialysis?

*Answers overleaf*

**405.** Because of modern therapy hypertension is now a much rarer cause of renal damage. It can cause sclerotic lesions of arterioles which cause narrowing of the vessels with ischaemia and atrophy (arteriolar nephrosclerosis) and it also causes glomerular sclerosis. These lesions lead to a reduced glomerular filtration rate, microscopic haematuria, proteinuria, and loss of concentrating power in the tubules. They also predispose to renal infection. In accelerated nephrosclerosis associated with malignant hypertension, fibrinoid necrosis of arterioles leads to further ischaemia and infarction with increasing renal insufficiency which, if untreated, leads to uraemia and death.

**406.** Normal individuals, especially if thin
Hypertrophy of single functioning kidney
Polycystic kidney
Amyloidosis
Nephrotic syndrome due to glomerulonephritis
Renal tumours
Hydronephrosis
Developmental anomalies
Abnormally sited kidney (e.g. pelvic kidney, transplanted kidney).

**407.** In a hypertensive patient the bruit may suggest significant renal artery stenosis which can be due to atheroma of the renal artery or, more rarely, fibromuscular hyperplasia.

**408.** Acute or chronic renal failure and removal of toxins or drugs, e.g. aspirin, after overdosage. Major indications for dialysis in renal failure are:
Hypercatabolic renal failure—blood urea rising more than 7 mmol/l per day
Rising blood urea greater than 80 mmol/l
Serum potassium greater than 6.5 mmol/l
Serum bicarbonate less than 12 mmol/l
Deterioration or bleeding
Weight gain, oedema
Hypernatraemia
Intractible renal hypertension
In fact, the main indication in chronic renal failure is when conservative measures no longer sustain a reasonable quality of life.

**409.** What are the common types of renal calculi?

**410.** You are called to see a postoperative patient who has not passed urine for 24 h; what do you do?

*Answers overleaf*

**409.** Calcium phosphate ⎫
Calcium oxalate ⎬ 75–85% of all stones
Struvite (MgNH₄PO₄) 10–15%
Uric acid 5– 8%
Cystine 1%

**410.** The most likely causes are that the patient is mildly dehydrated or just has not emptied his bladder—these are easily corrected—but it is always necessary to take a history and fully examine the patient, paying particular attention to the state of hydration, cardiac status, peripheral perfusion, blood pressure and whether the kidneys or bladder are palpable. Check fluid balance charts and drug charts (for nephrotoxic drugs). Examine any urine available for cells and casts and, if possible, send a specimen for microscopy and culture. Measure blood urea and electrolytes. All urine passed thereafter must be sent for urinary electrolyte estimations. If the patient is uraemic, it is necessary to consider whether the patient has pre-renal, post-renal, or acute reversible renal failure.

*Pre-renal failure*—may be caused by hypovolaemia of any cause, shock, impaired cardiac output, sepsis, drugs and should be treated by cautious fluid replacement, monitoring this against pulse, BP and JVP or CVP.

If the patient is sufficiently hydrated, frusemide 250 mg i.v. may induce a diuresis and prevent progression to acute tubular necrosis. If no diuresis, treat as for acute tubular necrosis.

*Post-renal failure*—is caused by obstruction to the urinary tract. If obstruction is at the bladder neck or distally, catheterize the patient and beware of postobstructive diuresis. If more proximal obstruction needs to be excluded, arrange an emergency I.V.P. or, if the uraemia is severe, isotope renogram. Whatever the site or cause of the obstruction an urgent urological opinion is necessary.

*Acute reversible renal failure*—is due to acute tubular necrosis which may be caused by any of the causes of prerenal or post-renal failure, toxins, drugs, haemolysis, rhabdomyolysis, eclampsia. A large dose of frusemide (250 mg i.v.) should be given if the patient is sufficiently hydrated, to induce a diuresis but if this fails, an acute renal failure regime is instituted.

**411.** What is the significance of pyuria?

**412.** Do you know of any antibiotics or antimicrobials that are nephrotoxic?

**413.** If you had to treat hypertension in a patient with chronic renal failure, which drugs might you use?

**414.** Are intravenous pyelograms ever dangerous?

*Answers overleaf*

**411.** Pyuria with significant growth of a single bacterial species suggests a urinary tract infection.

Pyuria with mixed growth suggests the possibility of an inadequately collected or contaminated specimen, therefore repeat MSU. If the repeat shows similar results treat as an infection.

Pyuria with no bacterial growth on the usual culture media should suggest the possibility of T.B., calculi or chronic pyelonephritis.

**412.** Cephalosporins
Aminoglycosides
Amphotericin B
Tetracyclines
Sulphonamides
Colistin and Polymyxin B.

**413.** Antihypertensive agents which do not significantly reduce renal blood flow, e.g. α-methyldopa, hydralazine, prazosin.

**414.** Yes, if the patient is allergic to the contrast media or if the patient is very dehydrated. The contrast media can cause tubular damage and acute tubular necrosis, especially in patients with multiple myeloma, and can precipitate pulmonary oedema.

**415.** Is proteinuria ever normal?

**416.** What is the significance of finding casts in the urine? List the various types.

**417.** Aminoaciduria, glycosuria, increased phosphate clearance and increased urate clearance leading to hypouricaemia are features of damage to what part of the nephron?

**418.** How would you treat a patient in acute renal failure who developed hyperkalaemia with a serum potassium of 7·0 mmol/l and ECG changes (widening of QRS complex with high peaked T waves)?

*Answers overleaf*

**415.** Up to 150 mg of protein in 24 h is excreted in the urine of normal subjects—and this level is often detected by Labstix or similar tests.

Sometimes, strenuous exercise, fever, exposure to cold, abdominal operation or severe skin eruptions can give rise to proteinuria and these situations should be excluded before embarking on detailed investigations. Transient or intermittent proteinuria is usually of no significance if urine microscopy and culture, plasma urea and electrolytes and creatinine clearance are within normal limits.

Orthostatic proteinuria, the passage of a small amount of protein when upright, is a benign condition and confirmed by obtaining a protein free urine sample voided immediately on waking.

**416.** The following casts may be found:

Hyaline—consist of Tamm–Horsfall mucoprotein; can be normal especially after marathon running, during febrile illnesses or after loop diuretic administration; otherwise are a feature of chronic renal disease.

Faintly granular—contain albumin, lipoprotein or immunoglobulin; have the same significance as hyaline casts.

Densely granular—always pathological; found in glomerulonephritis, amyloid, malignant hypertension.

Cellular—covered with tubular epithelial cells; thickly covered casts are typical of acute tubular necrosis.

Red cell—indicate glomerular bleeding as in acute nephritis.

White cell—uncommon; seen in acute pyelonephritis.

**417.** The renal tubule.

**418.** Give: 50 ml 10% calcium gluconate i.v. with ECG monitoring
100 ml 50% dextrose with 20 units soluble insulin i.v.
If acidotic give 50–100 mmol sodium bicarbonate.
If dialysis not available give 100 g calcium resonium rectally.

**419.** What are the main causes of chronic renal failure?

**420.** A patient with established renal failure is found to have a sudden increase in his already previously raised serum creatinine. What could cause this?

**421.** When renal function falls to below 10% of normal, renal substitution therapy may be indicated. What types of substitution therapy do you know?

**422.** What systemic diseases may be present with asymptomatic proteinuria?

**423.** A patient brings you a specimen of red coloured urine. What are the possible causes and how would you set about establishing them?

*Answers overleaf*

**419.** Glomerulonephritis
Polycystic disease
Diabetic nephropathy
Pyelonephritis
Hypertensive nephropathy
Analgesic nephropathy.

**420.** Uncontrolled hypertension
Urinary tract infection
Urinary tract obstruction
Dehydration
Nephrotoxic drugs
Congestive cardiac failure.

**421.** Haemodialysis—requires access to the circulation by shunt or fistula; must be performed 2–3 times each week for a total period of 8–30 h; may be performed at home or hospital.

Peritoneal dialysis—initially only performed in hospital but the technique of chronic ambulatory peritoneal dialysis (CAPD) allows mobility, and is available to many more patients.

Renal transplantation—from living related donor or cadaver

**422.** Diabetes mellitus
Amyloidosis
Gout
Hypertension
Systemic lupus erythematosus
Cadmium, lead or mercury poisoning.

**423.** Eating beetroot—check dietary history
Drugs, e.g. phenindione, rifampicin, desferrioxamine—check drug history
Haematuria—urine microscopy
Haemoglobinuria and myoglobinuria—urine tests for haemoglobin and myoglobin; examination of plasma colour (normal in myoglobinuria; red-brown in haemoglobinuria).
Porphyria—check urinary porphyrins.

**424.** List the causes of haematuria.

**425.** What is the nephrotic syndrome?

**426.** The nephrotic syndrome may occur secondarily to systemic diseases. List them.

**427.** What are the indications for a renal biopsy?

**424.** Renal and urinary tract neoplasms
Calculi
Urinary tract infections
Prostatic hypertrophy
Glomerulonephritis
Renal cysts
Tuberculosis.

Other less common causes include sickle-cell disease, analgesic nephropathy, renal infarction, bleeding disorders and anticoagulants, trauma and foreign bodies.

**425.** A syndrome characterized by albuminuria, hypoalbuminaemia, oedema (and also hypercholesterolaemia)—these abnormalities being direct or indirect consequences of excessive glomerular leakage of plasma proteins into the urine.

**426.** Connective tissue diseases, e.g. SLE, dermatomyositis or rheumatoid disease
Diabetes mellitus
Myeloma
Lymphoma
Carcinoma—bronchus, stomach, breast
Drugs—e.g. gold, penicillamine, mercury, probenecid, anti-venom, antitoxins, contrast media
Sarcoidosis
Amyloidosis
Infections—e.g. post-streptococcal glomerulonephritis, hepatitis B, infective endocarditis, infectious mononucleosis, malaria, syphilis, leprosy.

**427.** Proteinuria of more than 1·0 g/24 h
Unexplained renal failure in a patient with kidneys of normal size.
Haematuria not due to a lower urinary tract lesion in a patient with a normal IVP.
Systemic disease with an abnormal urinary sediment.
A renal homograft failure.

**428.** What radiological and related investigations are available for visualization of the urinary tract?

**429.** What drug(s) may be useful in the management of nocturnal enuresis in childhood?

*Answers overleaf*

**428.** Plain abdominal X-ray—to check for radio-opaque calculi and calcification.

Intravenous pyelogram.

Retrograde ureterography—for elucidating the site and nature of an obstruction.

Percutaneous renal puncture—to define and aspirate simple renal cysts.

Micturating cysto-urethrogram—to investigate possible vesico-ureteric reflux or bladder outflow obstruction and, in association with urodynamic studies, incontinence.

Renal arteriography and venography—to confirm the presence of renal neoplasms and in the investigation of undiagnosed haematuria.

Venography is used in renal vein thrombosis.

Ultrasound—especially to distinguish between solid masses and cystic lesions and in the investigation of hydronephrosis.

CT scanning—for tumours, especially in pelvis.

Radioisotope studies—particularly to investigate renal function, obstruction and renal perfusion.

**429.** Tricyclic antidepressants—with imipramine as the drug of choice. It should not be continued beyond 6 weeks if there is no improvement.

# Respiratory Medicine

**430.** What signs would you expect over a consolidated right lower lobe?

**431.** What are the signs of mediastinal shift and when might it occur?

**432.** Do you know the difference between vocal resonance and vocal fremitus?

**433.** What is the $FEV_1$?

**434.** What blood gas abnormalities would you expect to see in a severe exacerbation of chronic bronchitis?

**435.** List the bacteria which might cause pneumonic consolidation?

*Answers overleaf*

**430.** Reduced movement of the right lower chest posteriorly, increased tactile vocal fremitus, dull percussion note, bronchial breathing and increased vocal resonance with whispering pectoriloquy.

**431.** Tracheal deviation with displacement of the apex beat towards the side of the shift. Shift away from the lesion in pneumothorax, pleural effusion and haemo- or hydro-thorax; shift towards lesion in pulmonary collapse, fibrosis or pneumonectomy.

**432.** Vocal resonance is the perception with the stethoscope of voice sounds transmitted through the chest wall, whereas vocal fremitus is perception of the voice sounds with the hand on the chest wall.

**433.** $FEV_1$ (forced expiratory volume) is the volume exhaled in one second from the lung during forced expiration after deep inspiration.

**434.** $PaO_2$: reduced; $PaCO_2$: raised; pH: reduced (i.e. acidosis); standard bicarbonate: often normal in acute exacerbation—becomes raised in chronic ventilatory failure.

**435.** *Streptococcus pneumoniae* (pneumococcus)
*Staphylococcus aureus*
*Klebsiella pneumoniae*
Other coliforms
*Haemophilus influenzae*
*Streptococcus pyogenes*
*Legionella pneumophilia*
(*Mycobacterium tuberculosis*—in tuberculous bronchopneumonia).

**436.** What should you think of when a pneumonia fails to resolve as quickly as expected?

**437.** What are the complications of bacterial pneumonia?

**438.** What is a tuberculous primary complex in the chest?

**439.** What is the standard chemotherapy advised for pulmonary tuberculosis in Great Britain?

*Answers overleaf*

**436.** Organisms resistant to antibiotic therapy given.

Pneumonia caused by non-bacterial organisms, i.e. mycoplasma pneumoniae, viruses, *Chlamydia psittaci, Coxiella burnetii.* In patients with compromised immunity, think of pneumocystis pneumonia.

Some underlying pathological process, e.g. carcinoma, T.B., bronchial obstruction, bronchiectasis, depressed immunity, cystic fibrosis (children).

**437.** Pleural effusion/empyema
Atelectasis
Septicaemia
Lung abscess
Metastatic disease, e.g. abscess, arthritis, bacterial endocarditis
Pericarditis
Pulmonary fibrosis (late).

**438.** A manifestation of primary T.B. consisting of a focal site of initial infection, the Ghon focus, with enlargement of the draining hilar lymph nodes. On chest X-ray, the Ghon focus is not always visible but may be seen as a small opacity in the periphery of the lung field (usually subpleural) in the midzone. Hilar lymphadenopathy is always obvious radiologically.

**439.** Isoniazid 5 mg/kg/day
Ethambutol 25 mg/kg/day
Rifampicin 600 mg/day.

or

Isoniazid
Rifampicin
Streptomycin 0.75 g/day.

Triple therapy continues for 2 months after which isoniazid and rifampicin (or ethambutol) are continued for a further 7 months. Other regimes may be necessary because of drug toxicity or drug resistance.

**440.** How would you treat severe acute asthma?

**441.** What is farmer's lung?

**442.** What are the signs of hypercapnia?

*Answers overleaf*

**440.** Assess patient particularly regarding colour, respiratory rate, air entry, and pulse rate.

Humidified oxygen—high concentration, unless any evidence of chronic obstructive airways disease.

I.V. drip to maintain hydration.

Salbutamol 5 mg by nebulizer—repeat in 15 min if no effect; if effective continue 6–8 hourly; if ineffective, aminophylline 500 mg i.v. slowly—continue 40–60 mg/hour.

Start hydrocortisone 200 mg i.v. stat. and repeat 4 hourly; change to oral steroid therapy after 48 h.

Start broad-spectrum antibiotic if evidence of infection.

Check chest X-ray (especially looking for pneumothorax) and blood gases (looking for hypoxia and hypercapnia).

Avoid sedation.

Ventilate if continued deterioration. Danger signs: exhaustion, inability to cough, altered consciousness, rising temperature, rising $PCO_2$, tachycardia (N.B. can be caused by salbutamol).

**441.** An extrinsic allergic alveolitis caused by exposure of the lungs to fungal spores (*Micropolyspora faeni* or *Thermoactinomyces vulgaris*) in dust from mouldy hay or other plant products.

**442.** Confusion
Drowsiness
Warm peripheries
Bounding full volume (collapsing) pulse
Asterixis (flapping tremor of hands)
Papilloedema.

**443.** When does hypercapnia occur?

**444.** Explain the term 'pink puffer'.

**445.** Define chronic bronchitis.

**446.** What histological types of bronchial carcinoma are associated with cigarette smoking?

**447.** A patient complains of coughing up blood. Can you list the possible causes?

*Answers overleaf*

**443.** It is associated with hypoxia and is a manifestation of ventilatory failure, which is seen in:

> Chronic lung disease, especially chronic airways obstruction.
>
> Pure hypoventilation in patients with normal lungs, e.g.
> drug depression of respiratory centre
> brainstem abnormalities (e.g. haemorrhage, trauma)
> neuromuscular abnormalities (e.g. polio, Guillain–Barré syndrome)
> thoracic cage abnormalities (e.g. scoliosis)
> pharyngeal or tracheal stenosis
> Pickwickian syndrome (hypoventilation and obesity).

**444.** This describes patients with end-stage chronic obstructive airways disease (COAD) who are at the pure emphysema end of the COAD spectrum and who keep their $PO_2$ relatively normal by major respiratory effort. They eventually die of respiratory failure. The opposite type of patient is the blue bloater who is at the chronic bronchitis end of the COAD spectum and who is hypoxic, hypercapnic, cyanosed clinically and dies of cor pulmonale. N.B. Most patients with COAD have some features of both emphysema and chronic bronchitis.

**445.** Production of mucoid or mucopurulent sputum daily for 3 months or more in 2 consecutive years.

**446.** Squamous and oat (small) cell.

**447.** Important causes are:

> Pulmonary infarction
> Carcinoma of the bronchus
> Pneumonia
> Tuberculosis
> Bronchiectasis
> Benign bronchial neoplasms
> Trauma
> Lung abscess
> Pulmonary hypertension
> Left ventricular failure and mitral stenosis (more usually pink sputum).

**448.** What is a Pancoast tumour?

**449.** Is the prognosis of a bronchial adenocarcinoma without regional lymph node or distant metastases better than that of a squamous carcinoma?

**450.** List the important causes of diffuse pulmonary fibrosis.

**451.** What is bronchiectasis?

**452.** Can pulmonary disease cause finger clubbing?

**453.** Are expectorant drugs of value in pulmonary disease?

*Answers overleaf*

**448.** Carcinoma at the apex of the lung (usually but not always squamous). It has the propensity for early invasion of surrounding tissues, e.g. bone, pleura, chest wall, cervical sympathetic chain (causing Horner's syndrome), recurrent laryngeal nerve (causing vocal cord paralysis).

**449.** No. The 5-year survival for the adenocarcinoma after pneumonectomy is 35–40% whereas the 5-year survival for the squamous carcinoma after pneumonectomy is 40–50%. Survival in oat-cell carcinoma is always very poor with few if any 2-year survivors.

**450.** Sarcoidosis
Mineral dust disease (e.g. silicosis)
Allergic alveolitis
Fibrosing alveolitis
Collagen diseases (e.g. scleroderma, rheumatoid disease)
Post-irradiation
Oxygen toxicity
Chronic pulmonary oedema
Blast lung
Drugs (e.g. methotrexate, penicillamine)

**451.** Permanent abnormal dilatation of large bronchi as a result of destruction of elastic and muscular components of the bronchial wall. Symptoms result from chronic sepsis of the mucosa lining these dilated bronchi.

**452.** Yes; bronchial carcinoma, empyema, lung abscess, bronchiectasis, fibrosing alveolitis.

**453.** Expectorant drugs have little place in the treatment of pulmonary disease. Steam inhalation is probably as valuable as any of the expectorant drugs. However, expectorants which have a mucolytic action, (e.g. inhaled acetylcysteine) may be of value in patients with cystic fibrosis.

**454.** What is the antibiotic of choice in the treatment of pneumococcal pneumonia?

**455.** Do coal miners suffer from any particular lung disease?

**456.** How would you treat a patient with a pulmonary infarct?

**457.** What is the most common feature of sarcoidosis seen on chest X-ray?

**458.** When you aspirate fluid from the pleural cavity, what should you do with it?

*Answers overleaf*

**454.** Benzylpenicillin (penicillin G) is the drug of choice unless there is a history of penicillin sensitivity or the organisms are resistant (very rare)—Dose 300–600 mg i.m. q.d.s. When the patient is afebrile, change to amoxycillin 250 mg oral 8-hourly. The use of phenoxymethyl penicillin (penicillin V) is limited by its poor absorption.

Second choice drugs are erythromycin, co-trimoxazole or a cephalosporin.

**455.** Yes: pneumoconiosis, silicosis, Caplan's syndrome (massive pulmonary nodules in miners with rheumatoid disease). Miners commonly suffer from chronic obstructive airways disease and bronchial carcinoma but these are probably related to cigarette smoking rather than coal dust exposure.

**456.** Relieve pain and give oxygen.

Start anticoagulation—heparin 5000 u i.v. followed by daily i.v. infusion of 40 000 u. In mild cases, continue for 2–3 days; in more severe cases continue 7–10 days. Monitor activated PTT which should be 2–3 times normal. Start warfarin immediately in mild cases and 3 days before cessation of heparin in more severe cases.

Physiotherapy—may be difficult to do effectively in the presence of pleuritic chest pain.

Look for D.V.T.—if signs, support stockings or bandages to legs.

When patient improved, consider whether there are any risk factors or underlying causes for the embolism.

**457.** Bilateral hilar lymphadenopathy.

**458.** Measure the volume removed
Observe and record the colour and whether it is clear or cloudy
Send samples for microscopy (with gram stain)
        red and white cell count
        culture (including T.B. and fungi)
        cytology
        protein measurement.

In special circumstances, samples may need to be sent for measurement of L.D.H., amylase, glucose, $C_3$ and $C_4$ components of complement, A.N.F. and rheumatoid factor.

**459.** Define asthma.

**460.** What are the causes of pulmonary oedema?

**461.** Can you give an adult too much oxygen?

**462.** What is stridor and what does it signify?

*Answers overleaf*

**459.** Asthma is 'a disease characterized by variable dyspnoea due to widespread narrowing of intrapulmonary airways which varies over periods of time either spontaneously or as a result of treatment.' (Scadding, 1963).

**460.** Left ventricular failure
Mitral stenosis
Fluid overload as a result of i.v. therapy

However, do not forget other less common causes:
Acute infections, especially influenza
Inhalation of irritants, e.g. vomit, paraffin oil, chlorine
Post-pneumonectomy
Shock lung
Drugs, e.g. opiates
Acute proliferative glomerulonephritis.

**461.** Yes:
If the patient has chronic bronchitis with chronic hypercapnia, oxygen may lead to lowering of $PCO_2$ and inhibition of the patient's hypoxic respiratory drive. No more than 28% $O_2$ should be given.

High concentrations of inspired $O_2$ in any individual for more than 24 h can cause direct injury to the lung by unknown mechanisms leading to an adult equivalent of hyaline membrane disease. This is avoided by keeping inspired $O_2$ as low as possible to maintain adequate oxygenation and to give additional oxygen for the shortest possible time.

**462.** Stridor is a crowing sound on inspiration produced by narrowing of the larynx or the trachea. Tracheal stridor is lower pitched than laryngeal stridor. It is usually accompanied by dyspnoea, indicates serious airway narrowing and suggests the risk of rapid progress to complete obstruction.

**463.** What are the indications for tracheostomy in a patient with acute respiratory failure?

**464.** What lung diseases are associated with peripheral blood eosinophilia?

**465.** List some of the indications for bronchoscopy.

**466.** What drugs can cause bronchospasm?

**467.** Is sputum production ever normal?

*Answers overleaf*

**463.** To bypass an upper airway obstruction

To provide an entry to the lung for long-term artificial ventilation. Cuffed endotracheal tubes can lead to tracheal ulceration with tracheal stenosis if they remain in place for more than a week or so.

To facilitate removal of secretions.

**464.** Asthma

Allergic bronchopulmonary aspergillosis

Polyarteritis nodosa

Parasitic infections (eosinophilia associated with pulmonary inflammation during pulmonary migration phase of parasites such as ascaris, hookworm, filarial worms)

Loeffler's syndrome (eosinophilia and transient pulmonary infiltration).

**465.** Hilar mass

Haemoptysis

Pulmonary or lobar collapse

Suspected foreign body

Suspected bronchial tumour

Pneumonia that is slow to resolve

Retained secretions.

**466.** Asthma may be precipitated by β-blockers, tartrazine, aspirin, non-steroidal anti-inflammatory drugs, paracetamol, dextropropoxyphene, penicillin.

Bronchospasm as part of anaphylaxis can be caused by a wide variety of drugs, especially penicillin, streptomycin, iron-dextran, iodinated drugs or contrast media.

Acute bronchospasm may be induced by drugs releasing histamine, e.g. papaveretum, morphine, thiopentone, curare.

**467.** Sputum production is always abnormal. The healthy mucous glands of the respiratory tract produce about 100 ml secretion every 24 h nearly all of which is swallowed. Many smokers erroneously consider their morning phlegm as entirely normal!

**468.** Why is an occupational history important in a patient with respiratory disease?

**469.** In what respiratory conditions may skin tests be useful?

**470.** What are the indications for bronchography?

**471.** What organisms are usually incriminated in an acute exacerbation of chronic bronchitis?

**472.** What is cor pulmonale and how do you treat it?

*Answers overleaf*

**468.** Because the lungs are in constant contact with the environment and potentially at risk of meeting organic and inorganic pathogens especially in certain dust laden occupations. Examples include occupational asthma in epoxy resin workers, extrinsic allergic alveolitis in farmers and pneumoconiosis in coal miners.

**469.** Asthma—demonstration of cutaneous hypersensitivity is useful to classify a patient as having atopic asthma but only in a minority does it identify the offending allergen, e.g. aspergillus.

Sarcoidosis—the Kveim test is only positive in approximately 65% of cases.

Tuberculosis—the tuberculin test has limited value in the individual case but a positive reaction under the age of 5 years or a documented conversion from negative to positive at any age is an indication for treatment.

**470.** The main indication is to demonstrate a localized area of bronchiectasis, particularly if surgery is being considered. Identification of obstruction in distal bronchi sometimes requires bronchography.

**471.** *Haemophilis influenzae*
*Streptococcus pneumoniae.*

**472.** Cor pulmonale, or pulmonary heart disease is failure of the right ventricle as a result of parenchymal lung disease or primary disease of the pulmonary blood vessels. Chronic obstructive airways disease is the most important cause for cor pulmonale in the U.K.

Treatment is that of the underlying condition and recently attention has been drawn to the benefits of long-term continuous domiciliary oxygen therapy in 'blue and bloated' patients. In addition, treatment of the right heart failure is indicated with diuretics. High potency loop diuretics are used initially; spironolactone may need to be added. Digoxin is not thought useful in the absence of atrial fibrillation. Vasodilator therapy may be useful but further studies are needed. Venesection may be helpful if haematocrit is greater than 55%.

**473.** When is an antibiotic indicated in the treatment of a sore throat?

**474.** Name the non-bacterial organisms that cause primary atypical pneumonia.

**475.** What are the causes of pneumonia complicating influenza?

**476.** What is the incidence of cystic fibrosis?

**477.** What are the indications for surgery in bronchiectasis?

**478.** Give the differential diagnosis of cavitation on a chest X-ray.

**479.** What is Legionnaire's disease and why is it so called?

*Answers overleaf*

**473.** Rarely, as most sore throats are due to viral infections. If purulent tonsillitis (usually due to *Streptococcus pyogenes*) is seen, it would be reasonable to prescribe penicillin or erythromycin if the patient is sensitive to penicillin. Other causes include infectious mononucleosis, gonorrhoea, diphtheria and candida.

**474.** *Mycoplasma pneumoniae*
*Chlamydia psittaci* (psittacosis)
*Coxiella burnetii* (Q fever)
Viruses, especially influenza and chicken pox.

**475.** Only 20% of pneumonias in influenza are caused by the virus. The remainder are due to a variety of bacteria, especially staphylococcus and pneumococcus.

**476.** 1 : 2000 live births; autosomal recessive gene carried by 1 in 20 persons.

**477.** Localized disease leading to repeated infection or haemoptysis. Generalized airways obstruction and extensive disease are contraindications.

**478.** T.B., carcinoma, staphylococcal and klebsiella pneumonia, lung abscess, coccidioidomycosis, histoplasmosis.

**479.** Legionnaire's disease is pneumonia caused by a newly-recognized gram-negative rod, *Legionella pneumophilia*. The organism was first identified in 1976 after the severe outbreak of pneumonia at an American Legion Convention in Philadelphia, in which 29 out of 182 cases died. Serological techniques have demonstrated that this organism was responsible for previous outbreaks of severe respiratory illness, and serology with a rising titre of antibodies is the mainstay of diagnosis. Erythromycin has been shown to be the most effective treatment.

**480.** What factors are said to predispose to tuberculosis?

**481.** What are the different types of primary bronchial carcinoma and their relative frequency?

**482.** What diseases may be related to asbestos exposure?

**483.** What is the source of the antigens in bird fancier's lung?

**484.** What systemic disorders are associated with fibrosing alveolitis?

**485.** What is the differential diagnosis of bilateral hilar lymphadenopathy?

*Answers overleaf*

**480.** Previous partial or total gastrectomy
Diabetes mellitus
Steroid therapy and therapy with other immunosuppressives
Alcoholism
Silicosis
Malignancy
Malnutrition.

**481.** Squamous cell 60%
Large cell and oat cell 30%
Adenocarcinoma 10%
Alveolar cell 2%

**482.** Asbestosis—leads to diffuse pulmonary fibrosis. It is produced by
occupational exposure to any type of asbestos.
Bronchial carcinoma—complicates 50% cases of asbestosis.
Pleural mesothelioma—a malignant tumour developing 20–40 years
after occupational exposure to blue asbestos.
Pleural plaques—may become calcified.

**483.** Avian serum proteins, present in excreta and in dust from
feathers.

**484.** Connective tissue diseases, e.g. systemic lupus erythematosus,
progressive systemic sclerosis, rheumatoid arthritis, dermato-and
polymyositis.
Chronic active hepatitis
Renal tubular acidosis
Coeliac disease.

**485.** T.B., lymphoma, metastatic carcinoma, sarcoidosis, histoplasmosis,
coccidioidomycosis, berylliosis.

**486.** What are the physical signs of spontaneous pneumothorax?

Air in the pleural cavity

**487.** In what groups of patients does spontaneous pneumothorax occur?

**488.** How may a lung biopsy be obtained?

**489.** What tests are useful in identifying the offending allergens in allergic rhinitis?

*Answers overleaf*

**486.** Tachypnoea—if large or under tension

Poor expansion of chest

Mediastinal shift with trachea and apex displaced away from the affected side

Signs over the pneumothorax are hyperresonance to percussion, diminished breath sounds, reduced vocal fremitus and resonance and a positive coin sound (metallic sound heard on auscultation at front when coin is laid on posterior wall and struck with another).

Systolic clicking sound sometimes heard in a left-sided pneumothorax.

**487.** Most commonly it occurs in young healthy lean men due to the rupture of pleural bullae. It may also occur in middle-aged patients with a long history of respiratory illness usually chronic bronchitis or asthma. Rarely it may occur as a complication of other lung diseases capable of producing cavities such as bronchial carcinoma and staphylococcal pneumonia, or in connective-tissue diseases such as Marfan's syndrome.

**488.** With the aid of fibreoptic bronchoscopy, which has greatly increased the ease of access to the lung. It permits visualization of all segmental and subsegmental bronchi and the biopsy forceps can be extended beyond the tip of the bronchoscope permitting transbronchial lung biopsy. This has largely superseded the other closed methods of biopsy using either a cutting needle or drill technique. Open biopsy at thoracotomy is still sometimes required and is a relatively safe procedure, permitting direct visualization of the optimum biopsy site.

**489.** Nasal provocation tests which should be performed with care with very dilute solutions. Challenging the bronchi should be avoided by testing while the patient is in full inspiration.

Radio-allergosorbent tests (RAST) detect specific IgE in the patient's serum which react against suspected allergens.

Skin tests do not have very good clinical correlation.

**490.** What is pectus excavatum and what are the usual indications for surgery?

*Answers overleaf*

**490.** So-called funnel chest in which the body of the sternum is depressed towards the spine creating a hollow in the front of the chest. The indication for surgery is usually cosmetic, the condition rarely interfering significantly with cardiac or pulmonary function.

# Rheumatology and Immunology

**491.** What joints are most commonly involved in rheumatoid arthritis?

**492.** List the radiographical changes seen in a typical rheumatoid joint.

**493.** Rheumatoid arthritis (RA) is a systemic disease. What features may be present in the respiratory system?

**494.** What is Felty's syndrome?

**495.** What presenting features of rheumatoid arthritis are associated with poor prognosis?

**496.** What is the HLA antigen associated with ankylosing spondylitis and what percentage of patients have this? What percentage of the population with this HLA antigen develop ankylosing spondylitis?

**497.** What percentage of patients with psoriasis also suffer from psoriatic arthritis? What are the nail changes seen in association with psoriatic arthritis?

*Answers overleaf*

**491.** Proximal interphalangeal (PIP) and metacarpophalangeal (MCP) joints, the wrists, metatarsophalangeal (MTP) joints and knees. Less commonly involved joints include the elbows, shoulders, tarsus, ankles, hip and neck.

**492.** Juxta-articular osteoporosis
Loss of joint space due to damage of articular cartilage
Erosions of bone around joint space.

**493.** Pleurisy—28% patients with RA may have pleurisy and pleural effusions.

Rheumatoid nodules—which on X-ray may be confused with neoplasms. In patients with RA exposed to certain dusts, especially coal miners, nodules are accompanied by a massive fibrotic reaction. This is called Caplan's syndrome.

Fibrosing alveolitis. This starts in the lower lobes and gradually spreads upwards. Even without clinical features of RA, this condition may be associated with a positive rheumatoid factor.

Obliterative bronchiolitis—rare.

**494.** Seropositive rheumatoid arthritis in association with neutropenia and splenomegaly. These patients may also have marked lymphadenopathy and vasculitic leg ulcers.

**495.** Rheumatoid factor in high titre
Subcutaneous nodules
Bone erosions occurring early
Vasculitis
Other systemic manifestations.

**496.** HLA-B27, present in 96% of patients with ankylosing spondylitis. 1% of those carrying HLA-B27 develop ankylosing spondylitis.

**497.** 10%. Onycholysis, pitting of the nails, hyperkeratosis.

**498.** What joint problems are associated with inflammatory bowel disease?

**499.** What is Reiter's syndrome and in whom is the disorder most common?

**500.** What drugs, used in the treatment of rheumatoid arthritis, are thought to have a fundamental beneficial effect on the prognosis of the disease?

**501.** What are the indications for the use of such drugs in rheumatoid arthritis?

**502.** What are the reasons for avoiding systemic corticosteroids in patients with rheumatoid arthritis?

*Answers overleaf*

**498.** A non-destructive arthritis, of equal sex incidence, commonly presenting as a monoarthritis of the knee may occur and in ulcerative colitis is usually related to the activity of the bowel disease and is abolished by total colectomy. The response to bowel resection in Crohn's disease is more variable. There is an increased incidence of sacro-iliitis and ankylosing spondylitis in both conditions. These may antedate the bowel disease, follow an independent course and are not influenced by bowel resection.

**499.** Reiter's syndrome consists of an acute arthritis, conjunctivitis and urethritis. Other features include a scaly rash of the palms and soles (keratoderma blenorrhagica), tongue and mouth ulcers. It occurs 4–6 weeks after an attack of dysentery or sexual exposure to chlamydia. The disorder is most common in the 16–35 year age range and males are affected twenty times more than females.

**500.** Penicillamine, gold, immunosuppressive drugs, chloroquine.

**501.** Continued activity of disease despite 6 months treatment with non-steroidal anti-inflammatory drugs.
Progressive disease with developing deformities, occurrence of new erosions or restriction of joint movement.
Troublesome extra-articular features.

**502.** The doses which are usually required to control symptoms will lead to Cushing's syndrome with weight gain, osteoporosis, etc.
A dose which at first controls symptoms is often insufficient later.
Reduction of dosage is often very difficult.

**503.**   What is rheumatoid factor?

**504.**   List the main clinical features of systemic lupus erythematosus.

**505.**   What is the CRST syndrome?

*Answers overleaf*

**503.** Rheumatoid factor is antibody with specificity for antigenic determinants on the Fc fragment of IgG and when unqualified refers to immunoglobulins of the IgM class which are detected by standard laboratory tests. IgA and IgG rheumatoid factors also exist.

The presence of rheumatoid factor is strongly associated with a number of systemic features but their role in the aetiology of rheumatoid arthritis is as yet unclear.

**504.** Skin:     Butterfly rash on face
Vasculitic rash producing punctate erythema, especially around the nails
Alopecia
Photosensitive skin rashes.

Heart:     Pericarditis.

Joints:     Polyarthritis—rarely destructive.

Lungs:     Pleural effusions
Pleuritic chest pain.

CNS:     Involvement is common but widely varied clinical presentations include minor and major psychiatric problems, seizures, hemiparesis, and cranial nerve palsies.

Kidney:     Glomerulonephritis, nephrotic syndrome.

Blood:     Anaemia, thrombocytopenia.

**505.** A variant of progressive systemic sclerosis with Calcinosis, Raynaud's phenomenon, Sclerodactyly and Telangiectasia. In these patients the 'Esophagus' is usually involved leading to the term CREST.

**506.** What is amyloid?

**507.** List some of the disorders that might occur in atopic individuals.

**508.** What drugs suppress immune reactions?

**509.** What does a raised DNA binding signify?

*Answers overleaf*

**506.** It is an extracellular protein which appears eosinophilic and amorphous on light microscopy but EM shows it to be made up of fibrils. It is deposited in many different tissues in a variety of situations:

>Primary amyloidosis
>Amyloidosis secondary to multiple myeloma
>Amyloidosis secondary to chonic inflammatory or infectious diseases
>Various heredofamilial types of amyloidosis, e.g. familial Mediterranean fever.

There are two main types of amyloid:

>AL—related to immunoglobulin light chains and is seen in primary amyloidosis and in amyloidosis secondary to multiple myeloma

>AA—of unknown origin but is unrelated to immunoglobulin and is seen in secondary amyloidosis.

**507.** Asthma
Allergic rhinitis (hay fever)
Nasal polyps
Urticaria
Eczema
Anaphylaxis, especially to penicillin.

**508.** Adrenal corticosteroids—destroy lymphocytes
Cytotoxics and antimetabolites, e.g. azathioprine, cyclophosphamide—destroy immunologically competent cells
Cyclosporin A—inhibits lymphocyte multiplication
Antilymphocytic globulin

**509.** DNA binding of greater than 30% strongly suggests SLE and greater than 50% is virtually diagnostic. Occasional cases of discoid LE, chronic active hepatitis and Felty's syndrome have raised values.

**510.** List some of the diseases in which autoantibodies may be found.

**511.** What types of lymphocytes are present in peripheral blood?

**512.** What is multiple myeloma?

**513.** What is the commonest immune deficiency disorder?

*Answers overleaf*

**510.** Juvenile onset diabetes mellitus
Hashimoto's thyroiditis
Pernicious anaemia
Primary ovarian and testicular failure
Addison's disease
Idiopathic hypoparathyroidism
Idiopathic thrombocytopenic purpura
Autoimmune haemolytic anaemia
SLE and other connective-tissue diseases
Goodpasture's syndrome (glomerulonephritis and pulmonary haemorrhage)
Autoimmune liver disease (primary biliary cirrhosis; chronic active hepatitis)
Myasthenia gravis.

**511.** B-cells—15–20% of total count; are involved in humoral immunity and produce immunoglobulin.
T-cells—70–80%; are involved in cell-mediated immunity. There are various types functioning as helper, suppressor or cytotoxic effector cells in immune reactions.
Null cells—2–20%; are unidentifiable as T- or B-cells. Some may be undifferentiated T- or B- cells; others are K- (killer) cells involved in effecting antibody-dependent cell-mediated cytotoxicity.

**512.** A disseminated plasma cell neoplasm which causes bone destruction, hypercalcaemia and renal failure. A monoclonal band of abnormal immunoglobulin (IgA or IgG) produced by the myeloma cells is found in the blood on protein electrophoresis and immuloglobulin light chains are usually found in the urine (Bence Jones proteinuria).

**513.** Selective IgA deficiency; it occurs in about 1 in 600 of the population and is often benign although there is an association with atopy, autoimmune disease and coeliac disease. Some patients develop antibodies to IgA and can have anaphylaxis during blood transfusion.

**514.** How would you treat an anaphylactic reaction?

**515.** What joint diseases may be caused by crystal deposition?

**516.** Which joint is most commonly affected in gout?

**517.** What can precipitate an attack of gout?

*Answers overleaf*

**514.** Treatment is urgent if death is to be avoided.

Mild cases
> Adrenaline (1 : 1000) 0·2–0·5 ml s.c. and repeat every 3 min
> as necessary
> Antihistamine, e.g. chlorpheniramine 10 mg i.v.

Severe cases
> Oxygen
> Adrenaline i.v.
> Antihistamine i.v.
> Plasma expanders i.v.
> Pressor agents if patient is hypotensive
> Steroids i.v.—not effective immediately but are helpful if
> situation is severe enough to lead to persisting broncho-s
> pasm and hypotension.
> Bronchodilators and even ventilation if bronchospasm is
> severe.

**515.** Gout
Pseudogout (pyrophosphate arthropathy)
Osteoarthritis—hydroxyapatite may be found in some cases.

**516.** Metatarsophalangeal joint of the big toe.

**517.** Alcohol
Dietary excess
Starvation in obese patients
Trauma
Surgery
Vigorous diuresis by any means
Drugs—thiazides
> pyrazinamide
> uricosurics in low dose
> allopurinol (at start of therapy)
Chemotherapy of haematological malignancies.

**518.** How would you treat an acute attack of gout?

**519.** Why is early diagnosis and treatment of temporal arteritis vital?

**520.** What rheumatological disorder is frequently associated with temporal arteritis?

**521.** If you make a diagnosis of dermatomyositis, what underlying disease might be present?

*Answers overleaf*

**518.** The treatment of choice is indomethacin. Colchicine is an alternative; it is rapidly effective but the dose required may cause gastro-intestinal side effects, especially diarrhoea. It is useful diagnostically because it is only effective in gout. Phenylbutazone is no longer indicated because of the high risk of serious side effects. Long term therapy with allopurinol may be started 2–3 weeks after the acute attack has settled.

**519.** Because it can rapidly cause blindness; indeed blindness may be the presenting complaint. Steroid treatment is rapidly effective and prevents progression to blindness.

**520.** Polymyalgia rheumatica; the patient complains of pain and stiffness in the limb girdle muscles, especially in the mornings, associated with malaise and tiredness. Steroids are rapidly effective in treating the disorder.

**521.** Internal malignancy; 15–20% of adults with the disease have an underlying malignancy. The reason for the association is unknown.

# Index

*Numbers refer to Question numbers*